"BEAUTIFULLY TOLD AND INTENSELY INVOLVING . . . To watch another man seek after self-knowledge is to be reminded of our own moral duty to do likewise. By knowing others, we can learn how to know ourselves."

—*The Baltimore Sun*

"Deeply affecting . . . Unforgettable . . . Kondracke seems to be a natural truth-teller, and the directness of his narrative, its demotic lack of interest in irony when confronted with the rudimentary facts of mortal illness, opens his reader's heart and engages his reader's mind."

—*The New Republic*

"This is Morton Kondracke's account of his wife's battle with Parkinson's disease and his own transformation from a self-described careerist with more drive than talent to a *mensch* who has achieved greatness in this one book alone. I finished it last night in tears."

—RICHARD COHEN, *The Washington Post*

"Morton's love for Milly has been unfailingly strong and steadfast . . . in sickness and in health. His fierce devotion has inspired him to move mountains, and move scientists closer than ever to finding a cure for this cruel disease. We all must join together to fight for more money so we can save our most precious resource—the lives of those we love."

—KATIE COURIC

"Powerful . . . Kondracke pleads eloquently for Parkinson's research while telling a story almost too painful to read."

—*The New York Times Book Review*

"*Saving Milly* is a small but powerful memoir of Morton Kondracke's joys and sorrows, and a moving memorial to his wonderful but dying wife."

—*The Weekly Standard*

Please turn the page for more reviews. . . .

"THIS BOOK IS BRIMMING WITH COURAGE AND CANDOR."

—*The Hill*

"In a world where fast-cut video images too often dominate our connection to one another, Morton Kondracke creates a moving picture with his words of a life filled with human flaws, hard work, pain, hope, failure, and accomplishment—a life many of us recognize, made special by one constant, one great strength, his Milly. He reminds us, in poignant and very personal ways, of the power born from the passion of human relationships—passion that sustains us, that drives us to accomplish extraordinary things."

—MARY TYLER MOORE
International Chairman
Juvenile Diabetes Research Foundation

"Morton Kondracke's extraordinarily moving account of his marriage and his wife Milly's struggle with Parkinson's disease demonstrates how life's most difficult challenges can reorder our priorities in the most worthwhile ways. It also reminds us of the urgent necessity to increase funding for medical research."

—CHRISTOPHER REEVE

"[Kondracke's] confessions are honest and simple and ache with humanity. . . . In sickness and health, his marriage to Milly Martinez had a more profound impact on Morton Kondracke than he ever could have imagined. *Saving Milly* tells this inspiring story, and tells it truly."

—*The Oregonian*

"This book is a love letter, an involving story of the devastating impact of Parkinson's, and a polemic demanding a substantial increase in federal funds for medical research."

—*Booklist* (starred review)

"Their story is tender, loving, and funny—every couple's tale, yet uniquely their own. . . . Whether or not [a cure] comes in time for Milly, her husband has seen to it that her courage and wit will be long remembered."

—*Library Journal* (starred review)

Saving Milly

Saving Milly

Love, Politics,
and Parkinson's Disease

MORTON KONDRACKE

Ballantine Books • New York

For our daughters,
Alexandra and Andréa,

and our mothers,
Anita and Genevieve

Contents

Thanks

This book would not have been written had not Dr. Dorree Lynn, therapist and friend to both Milly and me, suggested that I needed to tell the world about our marriage and our joint struggle with Parkinson's disease. She not only convinced me to write it but put me in touch with her friend Barbara Feinman, who became my writing coach and cheerleader. Barbara's husband, Dennis Todd, suggested the title. And Barbara put me in touch with her friend Deborah Grosvenor, who, as my agent, also coached and cheered.

This book would not have been published—and might never have been written—had not Peter Osnos, publisher of Public Affairs and my long-ago Washington neighbor, friend, and journalistic colleague, believed from the first that the story should be told and could have an impact on public policy. My editor, Lisa Kaufman, said this was the most beautiful love letter she had ever read and, with copyeditor Cindy Buck and managing editor Robert Kimzey, turned a manuscript into a book. I'm grateful to

Tracy Brown, my editor at Ballantine, for his work on this paperback edition.

Many friends have helped in various ways, some by reading drafts and making suggestions, others by just being friends. Many of them are named in the book, including especially Jill Schuker, Mark and Judy Siegel, Terry Schaefer, Lori and Jerry Long, Terry Lierman, Fred Barnes, Jerry Leachman, David Bradley, Kathy Kemper, Gloria and Denis Doyle, Netty Graulich, Renee Gardner, and Alex and Paul Wheeler. Some who are not named include Ruth and Nick Daniloff, Sandy and Floss Frucher, Fred Graefe, Paul London and Paula Stern, Steve Rice, Barbara Barnes, Michelle Remillard, B. J. Frame, Jane MacLeish, and Dennis Doran.

Some of my dear friends in the Parkinson's movement read and sometimes corrected the manuscript, including Joan Samuelson, Mike Claeys, Ed Long, Danelle Black, and Michael J. Fox. So did two of Milly's doctors, Mahlon DeLong and Tom Chase, who made sure I got my science reasonably straight.

And I am grateful to my colleagues at *Roll Call* newspaper, Ed Henry, Tim Curran, Cindy Cunningham, Karen Whitman, and Laurie Battaglia-Skinker, who gave me encouragement and the time and infrastructure to write.

Foreword

The morning I testified before a Senate subcommittee in support of increased federal funding for Parkinson's research, Mort Kondracke did me the same great favor he is about to do for you: he introduced me to Milly.

I first met Mort just a week or so prior to the hearing. He had been among a small contingent from the Parkinson's Action Network who had flown to New York to prepare me for my testimony. When Joan Samuelson, PAN's founder, mentioned that Mort would be accompanying them, I was surprised and curious as to his connection to the cause.

"His wife has PD. He's very passionate."

Passionate? Mort Kondracke, passionate?

As a bit of a political junkie myself, I was familiar with Mort through his writing and work on *The McLaughlin Group,* and it was precisely his lack of passion, his steady unflappability in the midst of all the barbs and bombast that pass for political punditry, that I had always admired. Mort's appearance and demeanor at that preliminary briefing in my New York apartment supported this impression. Crisp and composed with inscrutable eyes blinking owlishly behind oversized glasses, his hair combed perfectly into a low sweep across his forehead, Mort remained a quiet observer much of the meeting. I had to fight the occasional juvenile impulse to tilt my head in his direction and in the manner of Dana Carvey channeling John McLaughlin bark out, "Over to you, Mor-TAHN!"

When he felt it was time to contribute to the discussion, Mort chimed in with obvious authority about the machinations of Washington, D.C., and specifically the politics of Parkinson's advocacy—who's helping us, who's hurting us, and who's holding us up by simply refusing to take a position. Historically, the PD community has been slighted when it comes time to disperse government research dollars, and Mort rattled off from memory the budget figures supporting this claim. Expressing sincere regret about my Parkinson's diagnosis, he nevertheless frankly and forthrightly strategized how best to convert my celebrity status into lobbying capital on Capitol Hill. Intelligent, illuminating, insightful, sitting there at my dining room table Mort Kondracke was also, in a word, passionate.

And so began my tutelage under Professor Kondracke, continuing in Washington on the morning of my appearance before the Senate Appropriations Subcommittee on Labor, Health and Human Services, and Education. As we wound our way through the literal corridors of power, Mort peppered me with information, pausing only to introduce me to this Senator, that committee member, and ultimately the Committee Chairman himself, Senator Arlen Specter. Amid a riot of flashbulbs I made my way into the crowded hearing room toward our panel's microphone-cluttered conference table. But Mort wasn't done with me yet. "There's one more person I want you to meet."

Cupping my elbow with one hand, locking it into place with the other, Mort shepherded me toward a bright-eyed, silver-haired woman seated in a wheelchair at the end of the first row. It was Milly. It is rare that a husband would introduce his wife to another man, a younger one at that, and then report with almost giddy satisfaction how instantly and profoundly the two were taken with each other. Mort sensed a strong and immediate connection, and he wasn't mistaken.

That first meeting initiated an exchange between Milly and me, a conversational thread that would be picked up over the course of subsequent encounters. Milly has inspired, encouraged, and commiserated with me. She has brought into sharper focus my personal understanding of such concepts as commitment, passion, dedication, suffering, perseverance, love, loyalty, and hope. Milly has taught me that one's dignity may be assaulted, vandalized, and cruelly mocked, but cannot be taken away unless it is surrendered. Physically weakened but possessed of a fierce inner strength, Milly Kondracke has weathered immeasurable loss, but that is one sacrifice she is not prepared to make.

What is truly remarkable is that Milly has shared so much with me without ever uttering one clearly audible word. Robbed of the freedom to express her ideas, feelings, and desires, she's bursting with all three. Milly's powerful presence combined with the depth of our common experience as Parkinson's patients accounts for her ability to communicate so much to me in the time we've spent together.

While prior to picking up this book you probably knew a little bit about me, and presumably something about Mort, it's a safe bet you knew nothing at all about Milly. Once you read her story, you'll never forget her.

At its core, this is a love story, poignantly told. Mort writes of his devotion to Milly with eloquence and surprising candor— from the more intimate details of their virginity-to-Viagra romance to the strengthening of his commitment as together they face the cataclysm of Parkinson's disease. Thank you, Mort, for *Saving Milly*, and thank you, Milly, for the love and passion you've inspired in others. I believe, as do you and Mort, that a cure for Parkinson's disease is very close, and in a very real way you've brought it that much closer. So who's saving whom?

Michael J. Fox
New York City, February 2001

Introduction

Parkinson's disease has kidnapped my wife. It is in the process of killing her. I hug and kiss what is left of her, hang photographs of the old, strong Milly throughout the house, and talk to her. We hold hands. We make love. But she is not who she was. She cannot walk, and now she can barely speak. She is being carried into an abyss, and I am helpless to rescue her.

I hate Parkinson's disease for what it has done to my beloved and is doing to one million other Americans. It is a horrible story I have to tell you, but it is also an inspiring one. For what I had and what I still have, I feel profound gratitude. Millicent Martinez was a poor, inner-city Chicago kid who grew up to be a dynamo. I wanted to marry an heiress from the Ivy League, but she was irresistible. Besides, I became convinced that God wanted this marriage to happen. So we married. Then we fought and loved each other in one way for twenty years and in quite another for the past fourteen.

Until she was forty-seven, Milly was always the master of her surroundings, the kind of woman whose will no bureaucrat, lazy tradesman, or alcoholic husband could resist. She saved Andréa, our younger daughter who's dyslexic, from being discarded by the school system. Andréa is now graduating from medical school at Johns Hopkins. Milly emptied my liquor bottles down the drain and railed until I went into AA, which changed my life and may have saved it.

Milly's Parkinson's diagnosis in 1988 shattered her confidence, but it did not stop her from fighting. A gifted psychotherapist who helped people remake their lives, she worked as long as she could. She underwent two daylong deep-brain operations, awake throughout. She importuned a president, testified before Congress, and cried in senators' offices to secure increased funding for Parkinson's research.

Her plight transformed me. From her resentful assistant, I became her dedicated partner. I came out of self-absorption and became an activist in the cause of medical research funding—not just for Parkinson's but for all diseases. I call that cause "God's work." It has heroes and heroines, and it is succeeding. If Congress and the president continue on the path of the past three years, they will double the budget of the National Institutes of Health. Then they should do it again.

Milly's disease nearly destroyed her trust in God. Until recently she felt that He was punishing her, but she did not know why. Parkinson's has had a different effect on my faith. I feel that I need to talk to God every day and ask for His help. Every time I have asked God what my job on earth is, the answer I've always received is, "Take care of Milly." But I cannot save her. If God can, He has not shown it.

Without God's intervention, a cure for Parkinson's will arrive too late to save Milly. Brain scientists say that enough is known that this disease could be cured in five to ten years—if adequate resources are devoted to the task. Despite the general increase in medical research funding, those resources are not yet going to Parkinson's. There is reason to hope this will change as my friend Michael J. Fox leads the struggle to secure research funding.

Virtually unable to swallow, Milly is now being sustained through a feeding tube. She can stay alive, but she is likely to be a prisoner in her body, able to understand but unable to communicate. She says, "I do not want to live this way, but I am afraid to die." I am terrified of losing her. I do not know how this story ends.

Saving Milly

"Marry Milly!"

"Marry Milly!" Joan Kehoe whispered in my ear. Then she repeated it, more insistently. We were at an Italian restaurant, Riccardo's, the favorite martini-lunch spot for reporters at the *Chicago Sun-Times* in the 1960s. This may have been the only dinner I ever had there. Joan had introduced me to Millicent Martinez a few months before. We were a fairly large and noisy group and Milly was sitting out of earshot as Joan importuned me. She also couldn't see the quizzical look on my face, which betrayed what was in my mind: *Marry Milly? Out of the question.*

Not that I didn't like her. I did. She was pretty. She was self-assured. And she was exotic, half-Mexican and half-Jewish. But she did not fit my life's plan, which was to become a big-shot Washington journalist. I figured that the person I planned to be someday should have a Vassar or Wellesley graduate for a wife, or possibly an heiress—a woman whose family connections and intellectually stimulating company could help me attain the goal.

Eventually Milly overwhelmed this stupid idea. Eventually I

realized that, wherever I went in life, I would regret it the whole way if she were not with me. So ultimately I followed Joan's advice. And thanks to that, I've lived a love story. But the decision took a while. And God had a hand in it.

In the first instance, though, Joan Smith, formerly Kehoe, deserves the credit. She eventually got a Ph.D. in sociology and went on to become a professor of women's studies and a dean at the University of Vermont. In 1964, though, Joan was an Irish American housewife and mother who was finishing college, abandoning her straitlaced cultural roots, and serving as spokesperson for the civil rights movement in Chicago. I was a fresh-faced twenty-five-year-old reporter for the *Sun-Times* who wanted to cover civil rights and politics—and meet women.

Originally I knew Joan just on the phone. She sounded so warm, I wanted to date her and was hugely disappointed to learn she was married—unhappily, as it turned out—and in her thirties. So we became friends. I sympathized strongly with the civil rights movement. The year before, one of my last assignments as a sergeant in U.S. Army Intelligence had been to watch the March on Washington and, if it turned violent, to meet up with troops waiting to be ferried in from nearby Fort Belvoir, Virginia. I listened to Dr. Martin Luther King's "I have a dream" speech with tears rolling down my face.

As a brand-new reporter, my main job was to write obituaries. I was ambitious, though. So, on a day off, I took it upon myself to knock on doors in a white ethnic neighborhood on the Southwest Side to try to understand why people there disliked blacks. They told me that they'd moved from other neighborhoods where, after the first blacks moved in, crime increased and property values collapsed. They alleged that the NAACP and crooked real estate dealers were in cahoots to spread panic.

Someone evidently thought I was from the NAACP and called the police, who called my boss, the city editor. He banned me from covering civil rights, though he let me cover politics.

Over the next couple of years, when I covered the Illinois legislature and then national politics, Joan fixed me up with various young women she knew. They included the first African American woman I ever dated and the first woman I ever slept with— the day after which occasion Joan sent me a congratulatory telegram.

In early 1966 she told me she wanted me to meet this friend of hers, Millicent Martinez. Given Joan's track record, I had every reason to think that Milly would be interesting and, possibly, sexually adventuresome. What Joan told me about her in arranging a dinner date sounded intriguing, too. She was the daughter of two Communists and, like Joan, was a student and anti-Vietnam activist at Chicago's left-wing Roosevelt University. Joan pronounced *Martinez* with the accent on the last syllable, not the second. Neither of us knew enough Spanish, or Hispanics, to get it right. In fact, for some months after I met Milly I kept mispronouncing her last name when I introduced her to people, including my parents. Finally she got fed up and corrected me.

Our first date took place at the famous Red Star Inn, a German place on Chicago's near-North Side that has since closed. Joan was a serious Marxist and yearned for a revolution in America, but her tastes were all upper-middle-class.

What struck me most about Millicent Martinez was that, at twenty-six, she already had a shock of white running along the part in her black hair. Even though Joan had arranged this dinner to fix us up, the dominant subject of the evening was that Joan was giddily in love and had to leave early to meet her new man, Larry Smith, a New York investment banker who was arriving for the weekend. Milly and I drove her to the railway station when we finished with dinner.

Afterward Milly and I went to an unromantic vinyl-and-Formica coffee shop near her apartment in Hyde Park on the South Side. Milly ordered tea. I got interested. *Her name is Millicent, and she drinks tea,* I thought. *This is a* classy *radical.* But it shortly became clear that she was less than radical. She told me that her pal Joan recently had enticed her into joining Students for a Democratic Society and participating in an antiwar sit-in at Roosevelt. Milly and others had been arrested, but Joan hadn't because she'd left the scene early to look after her children. Milly said she'd given the police a phony name, Rita Torrez, so she wouldn't have a record and could get a job as a probation counselor with the Cook County Juvenile Court when she graduated from Roosevelt in June. The police had discovered her real identity, though, and two members of Chicago's notorious intelligence unit, the "Red Squad," had come to visit her and tried to recruit her to inform on the SDS. She refused. One of them then sent her flowers and tried to call her for a date, she said, but she turned him down.

I was impressed by her personal involvement in matters I was, at best, only observing and writing about. I liked her politics—idealistic, but not rabidly ideological. She was on the executive committee of SDS, she said, but she was the conservative in the group, counseling others to keep demands reasonable and avoid confrontations with the police. She said that when one SDS radical brought a gun to a meeting, she had told him never to do it again. She told me that another guy's politics were so insane that he'd punched a businessman in the face on Michigan Avenue just for being a businessman.

I don't remember exactly what I told her about myself, but I must have tried to impress her with my achievements and ambitions. I was a Dartmouth graduate and now was jetting around the country writing about Lyndon Johnson's War on Poverty, urban race riots, and national politics and getting reasonably frequent front-page play in the newspaper. My ambition was to become a Washington or foreign correspondent. Milly was not bowled over. She clearly knew nothing about Ivy League colleges. The glamour of journalism did not seem to register with her either.

This definitely was not love at first sight, on either side. She considered me nothing more than "clean-cut." Even after we fell in love, I didn't consider her really beautiful, though when I look at pictures taken back then I can't imagine why. She was slender, olive-skinned, and sloe-eyed. She told me that she thought her nose was too big and her legs too skinny, and I guess I believed her.

But we were interested enough in each other—and respectful enough of Joan's recommendations—that we dated intermittently over the next few months. We went to movies, had dinner, visited Joan, and went window-shopping downtown—one of my favorite cheap things to do. I dated other women, too, including a Vassar graduate I fell into a maddeningly platonic relationship with. Milly was seeing two other men, a chemist and a professor at a junior college, both of whom wanted to marry her.

Even though this was the mid-1960s, the dawn of the sexual revolution, and even though I'd hoped that Milly might be a believer in free love, the reality was different. The best I got for weeks was a kiss good-night at her door, and a rather unpassionate one at that. She put her hands behind her—in her back pockets when she was wearing Levi's—leaned forward, and pecked.

At twenty-seven, I was ambivalent about sex. On the one

hand, I wanted it desperately and thought about it constantly. On the other hand, I just as desperately feared becoming seriously involved with anyone I wasn't prepared to marry. Moreover, I was ridiculously inexperienced. I was the product of a Victorian upbringing. I was a fat kid and rarely dated in high school. I was scared of women in college. And in 1966 I was still so caught up in 1950s behavior codes that I couldn't stand it any longer.

So I let women dictate the rules of engagement. If a woman was willing to neck, I'd gladly neck, sometimes till dawn. If, oh so rarely, one was willing to have sex, I'd gladly oblige when fear of commitment didn't get the best of me. Or, as with Milly, I'd accept the kiss-good-night routine.

After dating for a few months, we advanced to smooching. Once I decided to press my luck and clumsily planted my hand on the front of her shirt. She shot me a look that said, "Who said you could do that?" I blushed, laughed, and suggested we take a walk.

Since we didn't have sex early on, we talked. She had a fascinating story to tell. Her mother, Ida Lederman, had had a terrible childhood—she was sexually abused by her immigrant father and kept a virtual slave by her stepmother. She'd escaped by getting married to a Jewish artist. She left her first husband quickly and met Milly's father, Refugio Martinez, at a United Packinghouse Workers strike rally. Ida was beautiful as a young woman. Pictures remind you of Ava Gardner.

Refugio was a passionate, charismatic man with a sad, pockmarked face and prematurely white hair that he transmitted to his daughters. He'd prepared for the priesthood in Tampico, Mexico, but fled to the United States after being warned that his increasing involvement in radical politics was putting his life in danger.

Because his job as an organizer of meatpacking workers kept him moving around the country, Ida, Milly, and Milly's older sister, Alexandra, were left alone a lot. Ida was the victim of racial prejudice as an Anglo woman married to a Mexican. Once a brick was thrown through a window and nearly hit Alex in her crib. Ida later alleged that Refugio hit her when they fought and once kicked her in the stomach. They separated.

When Milly was three and Alex five, Ida suffered a nervous breakdown and ran away from home, leaving the girls unattended. They subsisted on breakfast cereal for a few days until neighbors called the police. Juvenile authorities found Alex outside their apartment building and took her to the Cook County youth detention facility, known as the Audy Home. Milly hid under a bed and was not discovered. She stayed with neighbors, who called for Refugio to come back to town. He got sole legal custody of them, and for a while they traveled with him, living in hotel rooms, until he placed them with another union organizer and his family in middle-class surroundings in Kansas City.

That family was unable to keep them, so Refugio transferred them to the care of Anita "Annie" Villarreal, a tiny woman with little money but a ferocious determination to improve her lot in life and that of other Mexican Americans. She had six children of her own and lived in a working-class neighborhood on Chicago's near-West Side. As a child, she had spent time at Hull House, the celebrated Chicago settlement, and knew its founder, Jane Addams, who urged her to stay in school. She was only able to finish two years of high school, but she absorbed Addams's social mission. She and Refugio Martinez were co-leaders of the Mexican Civic Committee, which helped neighborhood people solve their various problems, including dodging "the Immigration"—the

Immigration and Naturalization Service. Annie had been born in the United States. Martinez never became a U.S. citizen.

Milly and her sister were raised by Annie and her husband, Marshall, in poverty, but with strict Roman Catholic values. There were rats in the alley and bedbugs in the mattresses and walls of their house. The girls often felt the bugs crawling on their necks in school and crunched them in bed at night, leaving tiny blotches of blood on the sheets. Milly and her closest foster sister, Loretta (Lori), set off DDT bombs in their bedroom, soaking the walls with poison to kill the bugs. Milly believes that DDT is the cause of her Parkinson's disease. She may be right. Recent research shows that environmental toxins are significant in triggering Parkinson's and may account for the fact that the average age of onset is getting lower and lower.

Despite poverty, marital difficulty, and hospitalization for tuberculosis, Annie kept the family together and resisted Ida's desperate attempts to regain custody of Milly and Alex. She considered Ida unstable. Annie was a forceful, determined person with a fierce work ethic and Puritan values. Ultimately she earned a real estate license, opened her own business, bought and managed property, and became a local political power, twice serving as a delegate to the Democratic National Convention.

At a time when Hispanics are still woefully underrepresented on television and in movies, I have often thought that tiny Anita Villarreal should be the model for a series or a film portraying the upward struggle of Mexican Americans. Not only is she a strong matriarch, but her experiences and those of her children, grandchildren, and neighborhood acquaintances make a saga that covers nearly every imaginable sort of tragedy and triumph: forbidden love, botched abortion, infidelity and divorce, drug addiction, ethnic prejudice, upward mobility, political influence, bankruptcy, jail—and permanent family cohesion.

Somehow Annie managed to send all her kids to Catholic schools. The girls, including Milly, went to St. Mary's High School, where many Irish politicians and Mafia dons from all over Chicago sent their daughters. There were few Mexicans in the school, and once one of the nuns identified Milly at a school assembly as Jewish, causing a stunned hush. Nevertheless, Milly was a class officer.

When Milly was eight her father had a stroke. He was disabled and had to stop organizing. Nevertheless, he was pursued by the FBI and the Immigration and Naturalization Service as an alleged Communist. There is little question that his union was dominated by Communists, but his FBI file shows that the only proof the authorities could muster against Martinez himself was evidence that he'd once paid fifty cents' dues to a Communist Party front group. Nevertheless, the Immigration and Naturalization Service singled him out for deportation. His case, which is mentioned in I. F. Stone's history of the era, *The Haunted Fifties*, went all the way to the U.S. Supreme Court, but he lost.

Her father was deported when Milly was ten. She saw him for the last time through a gate at the railway station in Chicago when federal agents put him on a train for Mexico. He died within days of a heart attack. Milly described him as a powerful, generous, volatile figure who called her "Monkey" and had the smell of Camel cigarettes on his clothes when she crawled on his lap. She adored him. She told me that for years after he died she would imagine that he was in the room and that she would talk to him about things. It has always been mystifying to me how I managed to compete with that ghost.

Perhaps my advantage was that I was safe. By comparison with Refugio Martinez's life story, or even Milly's, mine was conventional and dull. My father, Matthew, was a salesman for a life insurance company no one has ever heard of. My mother, Genevieve, was a schoolteacher. They were Depression kids. My father's mother was a Polish immigrant scrubwoman at the Ambassador East Hotel, abandoned by her alcoholic husband. My father had a job as a bellhop there in high school. Once I stayed at the Ambassador East and made a speech in its famous Pump Room. I said, "Tell me America is not a great country."

My mother's family initially was more middle-class, but her father, a Jewish factory owner, died young and left my mother and her mother poor. My parents met in junior college in Chicago. My father went to work before he got his degree. My mother went to the University of Illinois, where her mother made ends meet by running a boardinghouse. My parents got married in 1936. They went on a delayed honeymoon the next year, eating peanut butter and crackers because they couldn't afford anything more.

By working tirelessly and saving, though, they made a comfortable middle-class life for themselves, my two brothers, and me. They loved golf and belonged to country clubs in Hamilton, Ohio, and Joliet, Illinois, where the insurance company sent them. While living in Hamilton, my mother got a master's degree in education at Miami University. My parents were apolitical but inculcated in us a disapproval of racial prejudice. The point was driven home when they moved to Springfield, Ohio, and were refused membership in a club because my mother's maiden name was Abrams. They were also loyal and dutiful. One of my brothers, Mike, was brain-damaged by an infection as an infant, and my parents set an example of caring that has to have influenced me when Milly got

Parkinson's. My parents rarely talked about God or religion. But our family did attend Presbyterian services every Sunday, and church youth groups always were the center of my social life, such as it was.

I spent much of my youth yearning to become somebody different from who I was. I grew up chubby, unathletic, and unattractive to girls. I was an above-average student, but never at the top of any class. A radio program, *The Big Story*, set the direction of my life. Journalists were depicted as heroes who saved innocent men from the electric chair or sent evil officials to prison. The show convinced me that journalism offered a romantic, exciting, important life. I started working on school papers.

At fifteen I got my first paying job for a real newspaper, covering high school and college sports for the *Joliet Herald-News*, and I worked one summer as assistant to the sports editor. This job gave me cachet in town and in my own family. My younger brother, Dave, was a state champion swimmer, and I humiliated myself trying to match him in the water. But my *Herald-News* job gave me the chance to shine at something. He could win a medal in a swim meet, but I was the one who made sure the world knew about it.

I desperately wanted to go east to college, believing that was the route to fame and sophistication. Beginning in my second year of high school, I began writing off for college catalogs, and by my senior year I must have had one of the largest collections in the country outside of guidance counselors' offices. Despite all my research, I applied to Dartmouth simply because another kid from Joliet had gone there. My father wanted me to go to the University of Illinois, become a doctor, and drive a Cadillac. My mother tried out the philosophy on me that it's better to be a big fish in a little pond than a little fish in a big pond. I said, "I want to be a big fish in a big pond." So my mother talked my father into sending me to Dartmouth.

In college I started out premed to please him, but ultimately I majored in English. Actually, I spent most of my college career working on the daily newspaper, *The Dartmouth*, known affectionately as *The Daily D*. I became its top editor but devoted so much time to (badly) managing it that I nearly did not graduate. I have little talent for making other people respond to my will, and I ended up doing most of the work on the newspaper myself. During summer vacations I got reporting jobs on small-town newspapers in Lebanon, New Hampshire, and Springfield, Ohio.

After college I enlisted in the army for three years to avoid the draft and in hopes of learning Russian or Chinese to prepare me to be a foreign correspondent. The army had other ideas, though, and so I served instead as an Army Intelligence investigator in Washington, D.C., doing low-level security background checks and working weekends at the old *Washington Star*. After my army stint I went to Chicago in 1963 to start my journalism career for real. During all this time I dated at most one or two girls long enough to have their mothers think the relationship might be serious. It never was. And sexually I had never been further than second base.

This was not a résumé designed to produce hubris. In retrospect, it's ridiculous that I thought myself superior to Milly. I had nothing to be snobbish about. The truth must be that I was unsure about my ability to achieve my ambitions on my own. I thought that the right wife might convince me and others that I belonged on a track "to the top," wherever that was. I was impressed in those days by wedding announcements in the *New York Times*, especially the first and last paragraphs. I thought mine ought to start, "Mr. and Mrs. Somebody Important announce the engagement of their daughter, ———, to Morton Kondracke . . . ," and conclude: "The bride is a graduate of Vassar College (or Smith, or Mount Holyoke, or Radcliffe). The groom, a graduate of Dartmouth College, is a reporter in the Washington bureau of the *New York Times*." I imagined another paragraph describing the bride's father or grandfather as maybe an ambassador, senator, or Supreme Court justice.

This wasn't just an inferiority complex married to snobbery. I had it on impeccable authority both that credentials count and that one's choice of spouse makes a big difference. I'd heard both things said by my hero, James Reston, a multiple Pulitzer Prize winner and then the Washington bureau chief of the *Times*. For years I carried his picture around in my wallet. When he came to deliver a major lecture at Dartmouth I heard him say that he believed people generally deserved the billing they had. I already thought titles were important. This made me do so all the more.

As editor of *The Daily D*, I summoned the courage to ask him to have breakfast the next morning at the Hanover Inn. There I naturally asked him how to make it in journalism. "Well," he started, "get jobs on small newspapers, work hard, and see who you marry." "That's so important?" somebody at the table asked. As if on cue, his wife, Sally, exited the inn outside our window. He said, "See that woman? If it hadn't been for her, I'd never be where I am today." The Reston dictum proved true for me, too, but it took me a long time to appreciate it.

I was impressed early on by Milly's grit and determination to triumph over adversity. Who could fail to be? Her mother was unstable, her father died tragically and young, and she grew up poor and had few peers who were going to college. Her sister Alex, finding the Villarreal home too rule-bound, had found a job and moved to the University of Chicago neighborhood. Milly followed and lived with her sister until Alex fell in love with an Englishman, Paul Wheeler, and moved to London. Milly took six years to get her degree, rising before dawn and making innumerable bus transfers to get to school and her part-time job.

I also appreciated that she had strong leadership talent. Her girlfriends in the old Mexican neighborhood organized a "gang"—really just a club whose members wore fake leather jackets—and their boyfriends formed a real gang called the Latin Dons. The Dons insisted that the girls be known as the Donettes. But Milly, the girls' president, decreed they would be called no such thing. So they became the Roulettes. Milly still stays in touch with a number of them. One of them told me years later that when another Roulette was raped, the first person she sought help from was Milly, who counseled her on how to tell her parents.

One of the other kids in the neighborhood told me that, as an artistically inclined, unathletic child, he was regularly hazed as a misfit. But he was defended and encouraged by Milly. She told him that reading was just as good as baseball, and she urged him to go to art school. He told me that, for years afterward, she was his model—for kindness, self-discipline, refusal ever to give up, and courage. Once when a group of Mexican kids was set upon by a bigger bunch of blacks, he said, Milly stayed with those who couldn't run away, offering to fight even though she was tiny and was razzed by her friends as "Skinny Minny." The confrontation dissolved, but what her friend remembers was her refusal to abandon anyone. Into adulthood, he said, "whenever I'd think something was too tough, I'd think, 'What would Milly do?' "

It was clear that Milly was a person with a talent for making friends. I didn't have this talent, and didn't understand it, but I admired it. Her roommate at the time, Andi Bacal, told me recently that part of it was that Milly was so genuinely supportive of people and attentive to them. Andi was a talented artist, and Milly made her feel more so. "Wherever we would go, Milly always told friends and strangers about her oh-so-gifted artist roommate. She encouraged, praised, and elevated my artistic endeavors like a mother would do with her daughter or someone blindly in love would do for her beloved. It wasn't until years later that I realized how unusual that was between women friends." Even though Milly had been poor and Andi was wealthy, it was Milly who told her roommate what clothes to buy to look stylish and elegant. Milly had impeccable taste.

It also impressed me that, unlike me, Milly was no respecter of rank, title, or authority. Early in our courtship I took her to a smoky, boozy *Sun-Times* staff party where the paper's editor, Emmett Dedmon, who was in his fifties, sat on a radiator holding forth on the errors of a major new book partly about Chicago, Jane Jacobs's *The Death and Life of Great American Cities.* Milly defended Jacobs's position through round after round of argument that left both Dedmon and me impressed by her spunk and command of the material. The more so in my case because I hadn't even read the book.

Even though Milly had gone to junior college and I had gone to Dartmouth, there were lots of books that she'd read and I hadn't, especially Russian and American novels and sociology classics. She knew more than I did about art, too, having been tutored, along with her sister, by an eccentric Hyde Park artist, Ernst Dreyfuss, a Holocaust survivor who allegedly served as the model for a character in one of Saul Bellow's Chicago stories. She was fluent in Spanish and subscribed to *I. F. Stone's Weekly* and the *New York Review of Books.* I had never heard of either.

All this aside, there were lots of things Milly lacked or didn't know about. I remember being mightily put off that she couldn't name the Democratic national chairman. Also, she occasionally used bad grammar. She'd say, "So-and-so is taller than me." I'd wince and think, *A Vassar girl would never say that.* She'd say, "We could go to the beach today. It's raining, but." I thought that construction was cute, and years later my heart would leap with nostalgic joy when she used it. In those days, however, her manner of speaking struck me as disqualifying in a wife.

Thankfully, she did not think herself disqualified. Quite the contrary. And more thankfully, though I did not want her, she decided to come after me, with Joan as her ally. Joan put the idea of marrying Milly in my head, even though I initially expelled it. Joan also advised Milly to use her sexual wiles. One day when we were kissing Milly stuck her tongue in my mouth. This time I reacted with shock. I accused her of being "forward." But shortly afterward one thing did lead to another, and we became "involved." Still, I remained uncommitted.

I dated other women and decided to conduct a little test. I was managing the *Sun-Times*'s election-year polling in 1966. In the pre-computer era this required meticulously calculating and recalculating statistics late into the night, using an adding machine. One night I'd have Milly help me, another night an Ivy League–educated lawyer I was seeing. Who did the numbers right? Milly did.

My heart fell in love with her one windy, chilly, late-fall Saturday in downtown Chicago. I remember the exact corner. I dropped Milly off to run an errand and drove a couple of times around the block, returning to pick her up. She was waiting at the corner of Randolph and Wabash looking for me, frowning in the sunlight. She was wearing a bright yellow raincoat, below which were protruding her skinny, spindly legs. She looked simultaneously intense and fragile. I found myself overwhelmed with warmth, tenderness, and joy.

I did not tell her that I loved her, though. I was afraid that if I did I would have to propose to her. But I couldn't marry Milly—she still did not fit in with my life's plan. I was smitten physically and emotionally. Milly's breath and mouth have a subtle, faint, unique smell and taste, vaguely smoky, vaguely metallic, to which I became addicted for life. Her hands are smooth and cool, and her grip is firm. Holding her hand is like being at home, secure. But my brain still was determined not to be in love with her.

She talked me into it. I was in her apartment, fidgeting with indecision, in a bad mood, in love but determined not to be. She demanded to know what was wrong. I refused to tell her. She said, "You can't keep your feelings locked up. What are you feeling? Talk!" I resisted. She persisted. Finally I told her that I cared about her a lot, loved being with her, didn't want to lose her, but didn't want to be pinned down.

I didn't admit right away that it was snobbery, but she wheedled everything out of me. And then she pounced. "You may know more about politics than me" (typical grammatical error), "but I know more than you'll ever know about people. I'm street-smart. I know how people feel. I know what they'll do. You may be from the suburbs, but you don't know anything about people."

I said to myself, *She is absolutely right.* This was one of the first of probably ten thousand arguments I've had with this woman over the years, and 95 percent of the time I've eventually had to admit she was right. I still did not say, "I love you," however. Instead, I started talking about the possibility of our getting married. I didn't propose. I'd say, "If we got married, we'd live in such-and-such a neighborhood," or I'd ask, "When we get married, should we keep your Volkswagen or mine?" If she dared to take up the theme, though, I'd get furious and accuse her of trying to force me into something.

It was time to run. In January 1967, I contrived a breakup. We went skiing somewhere near Chicago. She had hardly ever been skiing and was no great athlete. On a gentle slope she careened into me, screaming. I blew up and told her it was over between us. I justified it to myself: I wanted a woman who was at home in Aspen. I even told her I wanted to be with a Vassar graduate. Years later the one college Milly forbade our daughters to consider was Vassar.

We did not see each other for four months. We did have indirect contact, though. She was working at the Cook County Juvenile Court. Following in her father's footsteps, she tried to organize her fellow probation officers into a union. The group also sought reforms at the Audy Home, which Milly considered a cruel place to put homeless children. The chief judge fired everyone. Someone called me. I called a friend, State Representative (and future congressman and judge) Abner Mikva, who intervened with the judge and got them reinstated.

We met again on the afternoon of what I call "The Night." It was in May 1967, the first hot weekend of the year. I went to the Point, a spit of land jutting into Lake Michigan that serves as Hyde Park's prime beach. When I got there I saw Milly sitting with a bunch of people, including the junior college professor who wanted to marry her. I avoided her and sat at a distance on some rocks.

All of a sudden she was beside me. I tried to be cold, but within minutes I found myself agreeing to take her to the movies that night to see a double feature of Beatles reruns. When we got to the theater—the Clark, a grungy place that eventually closed down—I folded my arms tightly to avoid touching her. We talked a little, and lo, sitting immediately in front of us was Milly's former roommate, Andi Bacal, who'd witnessed our romance and breakup at close hand and sympathized utterly with Milly.

Andi swung around with an amazed look on her face and said, "What are you two doing together?" She told me years later that when she saw us she regretted that Milly was with me, afraid that her friend would get hurt again. But she insisted that, after the movies, we go to her place for dinner.

We went. We sat on the floor and drank wine by candlelight. We smoked a bit of marijuana. We laughed a lot. Milly and I emerged about 2:00 A.M. It was raining. Under an umbrella, under a street lamp, we started kissing. And kissing. And kissing. And I thought, *Okay, God, I give up.* Andi could not have been sitting in a crowded theater in the seat in front of us by any mortal prearrangement. This was a message I could not ignore. Years later I asked Milly why she had approached me on the beach. Wasn't she afraid I'd reject her? She said, "I loved you so much, I had to take a chance." That, too, was a gift from God.

I did not propose right away, however. I even thought once in a while that maybe I shouldn't. But three things made me. One, I had a haunting vision: if I didn't marry Milly, someday I'd be a Washington correspondent and I'd see Millicent Martinez walking around the Capitol with her husband, a U.S. senator, and I would shrivel inwardly and think to myself, *What a pitiful fool you are. You had a treasure—this strong, gutsy woman—and you threw it away.* This vision was entangled with a late-arriving mature notion on my part: if I did marry the daughter of Somebody Important and succeeded in my ambitions, how would I know it was my own doing? It was far better to marry the right woman for me, Millicent Martinez, and take our chances on what we could achieve together.

Second, I simply could not live the rest of my life remembering Milly's smell and taste and the strong way she held hands and know I would be without them. And third, Milly characteristically issued an ultimatum: you decide by I-won't-tell-you-when or we're through. Moreover, she said I had to ask Annie Villarreal for permission to marry her, so that I'd have to risk her family's wrath if I backed out.

I didn't back out. I did ask Annie. She gave her permission, although she tried to insist that we wait six months, as was appropriate for a nice Mexican girl. This we were not about to do. We spent the summer of 1967 not only planning our wedding but doing our usual thing politically and journalistically. Dr. Martin Luther King Jr. brought his civil rights campaign to Chicago that year, hoping to force Mayor Richard J. Daley into equalizing opportunities for African Americans. King led marches through white ethnic neighborhoods, including the one where I'd knocked on doors. The residents jeered at the marchers and threw rocks and bottles. Milly marched, risking bodily harm. I covered the events, relatively safer from injury.

We got married on October 7, 1967. We wrote our own wedding ceremony, praying for peace in the world and justice in America and also pledging in the traditional way that we would be there for each other in sickness and in health. Two photographers from the *Sun-Times* took different wedding pictures of us at separate moments leaving the church and walking to our reception. Both show Milly and me laughing, in a state of pure joy. I can't remember who said something funny, but I do remember that I finally felt utterly confident that I had made the best decision of my life. I have never for a moment regretted it, in health or in sickness.

2

The Old Milly

My favorite small example of Milly's old power unfolded on a steamy Friday afternoon in mid-August 1971. Massive thundershowers were threatening, and Washington, D.C., was getting ready to close down for the weekend and head for the beach. In fact, the next morning we were supposed to go to the beach for a week—me, Milly, our two little daughters, Alexandra and Andréa, then two and one, and our schnauzer, Tisha, three months. Our five-year-old Volkswagen Beetle, Milly's car during our courting days, had been in the shop for a week, and we'd been using the Volvo station wagon of some friends of ours, John and Lucy Masterman, who were out of town.

I was a correspondent for the *Chicago Sun-Times*, and I took off from work for an hour or so to cab it across town to the VW dealer, pick up our car, and bring it home for Milly to start packing. I had to get back to the office to finish a Sunday story, but halfway home the car's engine started hicking and coughing. The work definitely had not been done right. I doubted that the car would make it to the beach.

When I got home I told Milly that maybe we'd better use our friends' car instead. I assumed it was simply out of the question that we could get the VW fixed and retrieve it before the following Monday or Tuesday, when we were supposed to be away. Auto repair shops don't work late, especially on Fridays in August, and they don't work on Saturdays. I accepted that. I more or less always accepted other people's rules. Often I imputed rules to people when they didn't actually have them.

Milly didn't do this, ever. Immediately she said we couldn't use the Mastermans' car because they were coming back home the next week and would need it. In those days we couldn't afford to rent a car for a week. Milly had been a juvenile court probation officer before the kids were born, but now she was staying home for a while and not bringing in money. I'd just paid $400 to get our car repaired—that's $1,700 in today's money—and our bank account was nearly empty.

So Milly called the VW dealer. She asked for the service manager. I could hear only her end of the conversation, of course, but he obviously told her that if we brought the car back on Monday, he'd have somebody look at it. This is what I figured he would say. Had I been on the phone, I would have accepted it, although I might have yelled at him about what shitty work his place did and slammed down the receiver. That very likely would have guaranteed that the repairs wouldn't be completed until Wednesday or Thursday.

Milly didn't work that way. She said, "No, I have to have the car today. We're going on vacation." As I figured he would, he told her he was sorry.

"Who's in charge there? Who's in charge of the whole place?"

she asked. "I want to speak to him." She was transferred. "What is your name?" she asked. "Mr.———," she said, "I need your help. We are going on vacation tonight. We just paid $400 to have our car repaired, and it doesn't work right. We need the car. We can't drive it. It sputters."

Lo and behold, she got somewhere. The manager evidently said the shop would take it back for a look that day. She said, "Mr. ———, that's not good enough. It has to be fixed today. We need it. It was at your place for a week. We didn't have a car to use. We paid a lot of money, and it's your responsibility."

To my amazement, he agreed to have his people stay late if we'd get the car to him. I would gladly have driven it back, but she pressed on. "No," she said. "I have little kids, and my husband has to work. You have to send somebody to get the car."

By God, he agreed. But she didn't stop. "And you have to bring it back to my house when it's done. I don't have any way to come and get it." The manager capitulated. "Mr. ———," she said, "thank you. I really appreciate your help. You've saved our vacation. I'm very grateful. Good-bye."

This is the kind of thing Milly used to do in the old days. Milly ruled. She got her way. She never took no for an answer. Mostly people did as she wanted because they liked her so much. But, as in this case, sometimes she just made them. She was almost never offensive, but always assertive. I marveled at her power. Often I benefited from it. Her power was part of why I loved her. She was tough. I depended on her. But I was also envious and resentful.

The VW example is trivial. Andréa's dyslexia was not. In 1976 we moved from the District of Columbia to Chevy Chase, Maryland, because we wanted to send our kids to public schools but didn't trust the D.C. system.

In the fall Andréa started first grade. Upscale Montgomery County, Maryland, was starting a racial integration program, and she was bused to a newly reorganized school in a mixed neighborhood. As liberals, Milly and I were pleased with the plan. We were proud when a picture of Andréa talking with a little black girl appeared in the *Washington Post* the day after school opened. Unfortunately, the school's faculty and administration proved to have been selected more for public relations value than competence.

As tots, Alex and Andréa did everything early—walk, talk, tie their shoes, tell time. But when I tried to teach Andréa to read at three, as I'd done with Alex, she didn't get it. I taught phonics: "Cat is C-A-T, A-T sounds like 'at,' now try B-A-T." And so on. I was frustrated when Andréa couldn't do it. I got angry and yelled at the poor kid. I did things like that in those days. Milly told me to leave her alone, so I did.

Throughout first grade no one noticed that Andréa had a problem. The rule at Rosemary Hills School seemed to be that kids learn to read at different paces, and slower was no big deal. Andréa had a nice teacher, and she liked school.

But in the second grade everything changed. Andréa had a teacher—I'll call her Miss Smith—who was in her first year out of college. Miss Smith had a system: good readers got to sit on the floor in a circle around her, not-good readers had to stay at their little desks. Andréa is smart; she's now at Johns Hopkins University Medical School. In second grade she knew that she was being treated as a "dummy." Her classmates knew it, too, and she was taunted. She was humiliated and miserable. Some weeks into the school year she came home crying and said she hated school.

Milly and I went to see Miss Smith for a conference. "Some children are just slower than others," she said. It was a verdict I would have accepted. Had I been Andréa's sole parent, it could have had devastating lifetime consequences for my child. But Milly did not accept it. She insisted on seeing the principal.

The principal, Miss Smith, Milly, and I met. The principal, who was black, obviously had had experience with rich, pushy Chevy Chase parents who pressured their kids to achieve and tried to tell him how to run his school. He backed up his teacher and patronized us. "I know it's hard for some parents to accept that their children are not performing up to their expectations," he said. I felt intimidated by the fact that he was a professional educator and I was just a parent. Surely he knew what he was talking about.

Milly felt nothing of the kind. "Something is wrong here," she said. "Andréa is no dummy. I want her tested. And I want you to stop treating her like one of the dummies. She was happy in school last year. Now she hates it." The principal replied, "She has been tested. She is slow in reading." Milly said, "I don't know what kind of tests you are using. I know my child. She is no dummy. She is good in math. She learned how to tell time by herself. You have her sitting at a desk with the slow kids. Her friends think she's dumb. I want it to stop." This was one meeting that did not end with Milly getting her way. There was a chill in the air as we left.

In the car on the way home, we had a fight. I basically sided with the principal and accused Milly of being truculent and overbearing. She promptly became genuinely truculent with me, accusing me of failing to defend my daughter and taking the side of a beginning teacher and a damned-fool principal. "I spend more time with Andréa than you do," she said. "You're always off working. You barely see the kids. I know Andréa. She is a smart kid, just as smart as Alex. She learned to tie her shoes before Alex. She is just as good in math. If you won't stand up for your daughter, I will."

I was furious at being taunted and criticized for working hard. Milly was right about the fact that I was rarely home, but I was striving to break out of the pack as a Washington journalist, and for this, "enterprise" was essential. I'd been diligent enough as an investigative reporter for the *Chicago Sun-Times* that I proudly made Richard Nixon's "enemies list." I became the *Sun-Times's* White House correspondent, traveling constantly during the 1976 presidential campaign and doing freelance magazine articles on the side. Then I went to work for *The New Republic*, writing about foreign policy and traveling overseas whenever I could. Two times, for six weeks at a stretch, I went around the world from China to Vietnam to India to the Middle East to Europe, interviewing Indira Gandhi, King Hussein, and Yitzhak Rabin on the way.

I didn't think I was neglecting my family, though. As I angrily reminded Milly in the car, I always helped her write her papers for social work graduate school. I never went out drinking after work with other reporters and came right home instead of going to cocktail receptions. (I did my drinking at home, but that was only beginning to be a problem.) I took the kids to swim meets on Saturdays.

I had to admit, though, that she did know the girls' abilities better than I did. I also had to admit that she had an uncanny way of being right about things. What if she were right about Andréa? Even in the car going home, I felt ashamed that I would let the school write Andréa off and perhaps doom her academically and emotionally out of oversized respect for people in authority. Milly said that she would look for help. I said, fine.

Milly located a reading clinic at The American University and had Andréa tested. The verdict was: this child has a high IQ, but hasn't been taught to read. From being enraged at Milly's pushiness, I flipped to being enraged at the school's incompetence. We went to another meeting with the principal and Miss Smith. I spat out at them the judgment of the AU clinic. They responded, stubbornly, that Andréa *had* been taught to read, but she wasn't learning. The meeting ended with no resolution. Worse, Miss Smith took out reprisals against Andréa. It took more meetings to stop that. Milly resolved to find more help, including, possibly, shifting Andréa to a private school.

Somehow (with no help from Andréa's school) Milly discovered the Kingsbury Center, which specializes in helping kids with dyslexia. Andréa has a classic case of the disability, a brain circuit malfunction that scrambles letters. As we learned, it has nothing to do with IQ. Nelson Rockefeller, then vice president, was severely dyslexic and had everything on paper read to him. As we also learned, dyslexia can have devastating personal consequences. A juvenile judge whom Milly knew told her he was convinced that 90 percent of the delinquents he sent to jail were dyslexics who got turned off to school, were sometimes rejected by their parents, and started acting out and getting into trouble.

Andréa was saved—academically, emotionally, and professionally—by a Kingsbury tutor, Ellen Garfink, who began working with her in elementary school and stayed with her through high school. She was saved to an even greater degree by Milly, who fought year after year to educate the Montgomery County public school system, ostensibly one of the best in the country, about dyslexia. We looked at private schools, but most of them were no better equipped to educate Andréa than the public schools.

Eventually it helped that Congress passed the Americans with

Disabilities Act, requiring public schools to provide aid for handicapped kids. But Milly and I—principally Milly—still had to intervene to convince teachers and principals to allow Andréa extra time on tests, find taped books, and increase their understanding of the problem. Through college and into adulthood, Andréa had periodic nightmares about Miss Smith. Despite her achievements—art fellowships, top grades in premed courses, and acceptance at one of the country's best medical schools—she still isn't fully convinced that she isn't a dummy.

I am significantly to blame for this. For most of their childhood I treated her sister, Alex, who's more verbal and assertive, as smarter than Andréa. It's not true, of course, and Milly knew it. But Alex, now a filmmaker with a prize from Sundance, easily got into gifted-and-talented classes and advanced placement courses. Andréa made it sometimes, but not easily, and then usually because Milly fought for her. Alex would end up going to Dartmouth, where I had gone. Andréa got into Boston College, which, laudably, had a special program for dyslexics. Alex seemed destined from the beginning for some kind of celebrity. We all assumed that Andréa would end up a social worker like her mother—nothing to be ashamed of certainly, but not stardom. Eventually I would completely stop putting one daughter ahead of the other, but I admit that it took Andréa's astounding performance in premed and her later acceptance into Johns Hopkins to bring me around.

Throughout their upbringing Milly was Andréa's defender. She was the same for Alex. In 1973 I won a Nieman Fellowship to Harvard, and we moved to Cambridge. Arriving in the fall, we had a tough time finding nursery school slots for the girls, but finally we did. Within days Alex came home crying because boys in her class were being rough and disruptive. Milly visited, decided the teachers were not exercising enough control, and resolved to find another school. I figured this would be impossible and said, "Aw, leave her. She'll adjust." Of course, Milly soon talked the ideal school into making a slot for Alex.

Throughout their childhood she was the girls' primary parent and builder of values. I pushed grades, hard work, and getting into good colleges. Milly counseled friendship and made our house a welcome place for the girls' schoolmates. One night in the early 1980s, as Alex and Andréa were reaching adolescence, Milly convened a meeting of twenty or so parents in our living room and said that they all should help one another cope with the challenges that lay ahead—alcohol, drugs, parties, dating, sex, driving, and so on. She created a parents' information network (or "spy network," as the kids charged) to keep track of what was going on.

Our girls—and often their friends—confided in Milly because she was open and loving and genuinely interested. And also because she almost always knew what was going on anyway. Once Milly found out that a friend's son, a junior in high school, planned to deflower his girlfriend, just a freshman, while his mother was out of the house at work. Milly tipped off the mother, who stayed home sick that day. This strategy only postponed the inevitable, however.

Milly set the rules for the girls. I was always confused about whether to say yes or no to one request or another. Stay out late? Stay at so-and-so's house overnight? Can boys be in the house when we're not home? Even if Milly's rules were arbitrary, they were decisive. The decree was: "No boys allowed on the second floor." Milly was infamous among Chevy Chase kids as a rule-maker, but parents constantly called up for advice on how to do it. I marveled at her authority. I knew that, had it been up to me, my kids would have been out of control, since I would have just ineffectually yelled at them to do their homework and get good grades.

In later years Alex and Andréa delighted in trying to shock us by revealing that Milly's control system was not perfect. When they were teenagers they'd waited for us to fall asleep and sneaked out of the house to meet friends or drive our car around town. They drank beer and smoked some pot in spite of Milly's rule that when they got home they had to kiss her good-night so she could smell their breath and clothes. Boys did make it to the second floor when we weren't home—although there are no reports that they got to do anything there except talk. They certainly knew the rule. Once when Milly and I came home unexpectedly, we heard what sounded like a cattle stampede down the stairs as we approached the front door. We found a whole group of kids inside, boys and girls. The boys sheepishly apologized to Milly and assured her nothing had happened. Evidently they feared banishment from our house, which they valued as a haven. It wouldn't have happened because Milly loved having our kids' friends over. But she definitely commanded respect.

Milly also disciplined me. Once we went on a driving trip through Portugal and Spain. The girls were eleven and ten and seemingly had to stop every twenty kilometers to go to the bathroom. There weren't any rest stops. We had to locate a restaurant and negotiate use of the WC. In Portugal one day I simply refused to stop. The kids pleaded. Milly shouted. I drove. Finally she opened the passenger door and said, "If you don't stop right away, I'm jumping out." I feared she really would. I stopped. I apologized. I ceased complaining when we stopped other times. It made for a great trip. We read Michener's *Iberia* and Ernest Hemingway to each other as we went.

The Iberia trip was one of Milly's projects. She always had a project. A cross-country drive to visit her old roommate, Andi, in San Diego. A new dining room set. Painting the bedroom. New bedroom furniture. Remodeling the house. A trip to Chicago to visit her family. Moving her aging mother, Ida, to Washington and helping her buy an apartment. The projects invariably involved spending money, so I resisted. I had absorbed the Depression mentality of my parents. Milly, who'd known real poverty, believed that money was meant to be spent. When I discovered this attitude of hers early in our marriage I joked that she was a "Mercedes girl," though it wasn't until 1999, when she was badly disabled by Parkinson's, that we finally bought a Mercedes.

I resented the constant pressure of her projects, the drain on our bank account, the disruption of the status quo. There was never a respite. I'd yell. I'd bargain: "Okay, *this* time, but we're not spending any money for the rest of the year!" Invariably, she'd prevail. She was gifted at argumentation. She was relentless. By the time I yielded, she had convinced me that we really ought to have or do what she wanted, and that we could afford it. We did save enough money to put a major addition on our house and put our kids through college, but we also accumulated a heap of credit card debt. I fret about it yet. Milly's favorite recreation still is to look through mail-order catalogs with her Visa card at the ready.

I was not a total pushover. I imposed my will on big decisions, such as the houses and cars we bought. I don't bargain well, and some of the cars I picked were overpriced lemons, but they were my choices. I did much better with the houses, first in Northwest Washington and then in Chevy Chase. I loved them both at first sight, decided they were within our budget, and slapped down a contract on them within hours of seeing them, dragging Milly into the decision. In time she would agree that I'd made good decisions. The Chevy Chase house had a deep, beautifully landscaped backyard as its main attraction. Ultimately we remodeled, building an ultra-modern kitchen and wide deck with a view of the yard and the trees. The house was a joy to both of us and our children. Milly cried when Parkinson's disease forced us to leave it.

People, even more than projects, were Milly's great calling. She was a magnet for them. She was utterly democratic in making friends, and people attached themselves to her for life. When we first arrived in Washington we lived in a big apartment building at 4000 Tunlaw Road, NW, where the original rent was $149 a month. One day the management abruptly raised it to $170. Milly decided to organize a rent strike. She went door to door, got to know practically everybody in the building, and called a meeting in a church basement. The next thing I knew I was the president of a tenants' association and we had a lawyer, an escrow bank account, and a cause. A congressman lived in the building, and he gave us clout and publicity. By God, we forced a rollback.

Milly made permanent friends with some of the wives in the building and saw many through various hardships. One woman had an abusive husband and, some years after we'd all moved away to houses, finally decided to leave him. But she was afraid. So Milly organized the Tunlaw wives into a task force that swept into her house one Saturday when the husband was running an errand. They collected all the belongings of the wife and her kids into plastic garbage bags and hustled them into cars. They made a narrow escape, whisking the wife and kids to a safe place just as the husband drove onto his block. He quickly figured out who'd organized this and came to our house looking for his family. I told him that his marriage was over and that he'd best back off.

Milly made friends with people utterly regardless of their station. A hairdresser. A masseuse. A Sears repairman. A piano teacher. A sewing teacher. An artist. An English instructor. Fellow psychotherapists. Milly's best friend—virtually her surrogate sister, and mine—is Jill Schuker, whom we met at a party in 1968, just after we moved to Washington. Jill and Milly, who look like sisters, started working together on Robert F. Kennedy's presidential campaign and became soulmates for life. Over the years, as Jill moved from congressional aide to State Department and White House official to high-powered PR woman, she and Milly talked almost daily about everything in their lives, happy or sad. Jill's friends became our primary social circle. Jill has been Milly's most regular confidante in her struggle with Parkinson's.

Some other friends are almost as close. Netty Graulich, once a sewing teacher to the female social stars of Washington, helped Milly organize the rescue of their friend from her husband. Terry Schaefer, a teacher who became an NBC *Today Show* producer, was part of the Chevy Chase parents' "spy network." I have learned from watching Milly and her friends share joy and woe that love is like a bank account. When much is put in, much is there to be drawn out.

I understood this theoretically but was somehow handicapped as a friend-maker. I was intimidated by almost anyone I believed to be above my status, or smarter or more famous than I was. And I was snobbishly dismissive of those below me. There was a tiny sliver of people I considered peers. But I often got turned off by some trait or action of theirs or thought I was failing to live up to their expectations, so I rarely stayed close to anyone for long. Unlike Milly, I have no close friends from high school, college, or my Chicago days. Early in my Washington career I was chums with some of the future notables of American journalism—Bob

Woodward, Carl Bernstein, Tom Brokaw, Sally Quinn. But as they ascended I failed to stay connected to them, figuring they'd bypassed me. Fortunately, a few people insisted on staying close to me—often because they liked the combination of Milly and me. Had it been up to me alone, I surely would have lost them, too.

One couple we've been friends with all along are Mark and Judy Siegel, who moved to Chevy Chase to be our neighbors and followed us back to downtown Washington when Milly's illness forced us to buy an apartment. In the 1970s Mark was executive director of the Democratic National Committee and a good news source. I invited them to a party at our house as the Watergate scandal was unfolding. Judy was impressed with the company—including Woodward and Bernstein—but more so with Milly, who had cooked Mexican food for sixty people and yet had dressed our little girls charmingly and was available for conversation. Over the years Milly and Judy became child-rearing allies and co-skeptics about Washington mores, especially the tendency to judge people by their titles and discard them when they hit a downslope. We and the Siegels have considered each other's kids almost like our own. When Judy's mother died of cancer, Judy sent her older daughter, Rebecca, to Milly for comfort. Milly asked Rebecca what she'd been doing at the time her grandma died. Rebecca said she'd been taking a test in school. "What grade did you get?" Milly asked. Rebecca told her, "An A." Milly said, "That was your grandmother's last gift to you." The grade had actually been a C, but Rebecca still remembers Milly's remark for the solace it gave her.

We spend every Thanksgiving with the Siegels—formerly at our house, now at theirs—often joined by as many as thirty people, including stray college students and others without families in Washington. Milly, in her inimitable way, early on established rules for this event that became traditions: children sit mixed in with adults and are included in conversations. And after a prayer and before we can eat, each person says what he or she has to be thankful for that year. For years, besides the love and successes of our children, we and the Siegels and Jill Schuker have been saying thanks for the friendship of our families.

In truth, though, for many years Milly was not only my best friend but my only friend. She was the one person I truly confided in. She was the only person, other than my children, whom I truly cared about. We talked about everything—my career, my envy of smarter and more successful journalists, politics, people we liked and didn't like, money, her clients, our kids, their friends, our relatives. We talked constantly and volubly. Sometimes we'd go to other people's houses and I would talk only to her, even across the dinner table. Some friends found this passionate and exciting. Milly usually told me it was embarrassing and inconsiderate of others.

Had it not been for Milly, I would have remained estranged from my own brother. Growing up, David was a star athlete. I, three years older, was a better student and then a sports reporter. I was envious of him, and he of me. For more than ten years, from the time I went to college in 1956 until after Milly and I were married, my brother and I rarely talked—and when we did it was mainly to jibe at each other. One day, using her social work skills, Milly insisted that we talk out our differences in detail. When we got stuck or were obviously concealing something, she yelled, "Out with it! Tell him how you feel!" It took several hours, but it worked. We're not as close as brothers should be, but he's my stockbroker and financial adviser.

Milly was a gifted, natural-born social worker. Whether they were paying her or not, she listened to people intently, understood what they really were saying, and pulled out of them what they feared to utter. She violated the rules of psychotherapy by talking about her clients, though not by name, and I was always impressed by the progress she made with them. She counseled one unhappy man out of a gay lifestyle, and years later he still sends Milly letters of thanks with pictures of his wife and children. She counseled another deeply troubled young woman into accepting her homosexuality, and that former client also writes regularly, enclosing pictures of her partner and their adopted child. Milly saved marriages and helped other miserable couples separate amicably. She helped people change careers and taught lonely singles how to date. One geeky political aide became a champion ballroom dancer under Milly's influence, though he never did marry. Milly was always available to her clients by phone and rarely charged them if they missed appointments.

To Milly, status meant nothing. She became close friends with our Bolivian housekeeper as well as with the wife of Washington's premier sports entrepreneur. She was a pal and confidante of people on our block and of some in high places. When we went to a glitzy party she'd invariably learn everything there was to know about her dinner partner's family woes. On the way home I was always amazed to learn what she'd found out. I had usually just had sterile conversations comparing résumés and political views. Sometimes the people Milly met this way would become her clients in therapy. Sometimes they just called her for advice. She remembered them, and they remembered her. I, on the other hand, still go deaf when someone tells me his or her name. Even though I try to be pleasant and attentive to people, often I forget I've ever met them.

Milly's ability to get people to talk struck me as magical. It was unlike anything I had ever witnessed or practiced in journalism.

She never quizzed or pumped people. She didn't have to. She was like a powerful magnet for personal secrets. Friends like Jill Schuker and Judy Siegel say the key to it was that people knew she genuinely cared about them and gave them complete attention. What some people, especially men, might dismiss as gossip— love lost and found, jealousy and anger, children succeeding or having troubles—Milly understood to be the essence of life. She had nearly limitless patience and seemed to consider no one's feelings unimportant or beneath her interest. She was always available for talk, even if her friends had to follow her around the house as she made dinner or took care of children. She was hard to shock and slow to render judgments.

On the other hand, she was no fool and was invariably direct with her advice and opinions. If she thought someone was being cruel or dishonest, she told them so. If she thought they were covering up their true feelings, she punched through the facade. In the 1970s the *Washington Post* columnist Richard Cohen asked Milly at a party what she did. When she told him she was taking care of her children and saw him looking around for someone more interesting to talk to, she backed him into a kitchen corner and delivered a lecture about the importance of child-rearing. He wrote a confessional column about the encounter in the newspaper.

If Milly could talk to big shots and little people with equal empathy and interest, she had nothing but derision for my fear of using my connections and my tendency to underrate my influence. Sometime after I became the *Sun-Times's* White House correspondent in 1975, we were invited to a state dinner. It was rainy and cold, and when I started looking for a parking space on the street Milly said surely we were expected to park on the White House grounds. Somehow I couldn't believe we would have such a privilege. I finally found a space several blocks away. When we arrived inside, soaked, we discovered that Milly was right, of course. It was years before she forgot about it.

Late in the 1976 presidential campaign she got me into a memorable caper. Some months earlier one of her friends, a teacher of English as a second language, had fallen in love with a visiting Bulgarian poet and created a neighborhood scandal by leaving her husband, even though the poet had returned to his homeland. Then one day in late October Milly was on the phone to me on the campaign trail, telling me I had to help rescue the poet, who was in London and wanted to defect but was terrified he'd be nabbed or even killed by Bulgarian security agents. *Oh God*, I thought, *this Milly project is beyond the pale.* I tried to tell her there was nothing I could do to help him, but she said, "You're a White House correspondent. You're with the president! You've got to talk to somebody." I was getting treated like the VW manager. Like him, I buckled.

I called Milly's friend, who was petrified because of a recent, highly publicized case: a Bulgarian secret police agent, using poison in an umbrella tip, had murdered a Bulgarian dissident, Georgi Markov, on a train platform in London. The poet had ducked out of an academic conference and was hiding at a YMCA residence, but he knew no one in London, he had little money, and it was a weekend. He had called the U.S. embassy, but it was closed, and he had been told to call back on Monday. "Milly said you could help," her friend said. I went to a deputy White House press secretary, who said there was nothing he could do, that this was a matter for the embassy in London.

From a hotel room somewhere on the campaign trail I called Milly's sister and some other friends in London. They couldn't help. I reached the terrified poet and told him he'd just have to lie low until Monday. Then a bureaucratic nightmare unfolded. U.S. immigration officials told me on Monday that it might take weeks to process his appeal for asylum, and that he would have to come into the embassy to file it. He was terrified to do this, assuming the Bulgarians would see him and grab him when he came out of hiding.

A wild week ensued. President Ford was flying at a furious pace around the country in a close race with Jimmy Carter, and I had to cover three or four rallies, parades, and speeches a day. At pay phones and in pressrooms along the way I used my credit card to call London. I called the U.S. ambassador, Anne Armstrong, and she said she'd put an assistant on the case. Later the assistant said the Bulgarian's case was in the hands of the Immigration and Naturalization Service, whose rules had to be followed. I told the poet he'd have to summon his courage and go to the embassy. He did, filed his papers, and was told: stay in touch. I called the ambassador's assistant and INS daily to track the case and was told to be patient. I called the poet two or three times a day to check on his mood and safety; he sounded more and more panicky. Milly's friend, too, sounded panicky. Milly wasn't panicky, just insistent that she expected me to save this guy.

As the days went by I pleaded more urgently with the embassy, with INS, and finally with the White House's deputy national security adviser, Bill Hyland, that this defector was in danger of getting killed. "Remember Markov," I pleaded. The White House called the embassy, which confirmed that it knew about the case but repeated that it was in the hands of INS and there was nothing anyone else could do.

Finally, on the Friday before the election, I did what Milly probably would have done at the outset. I went to Hyland with a story I largely made up: "My editors are very interested in this case," I said. "I write for the *Chicago Sun-Times*, as you know. Illinois is a key swing state in this election. There are hundreds of thousands of Eastern European ethnic voters in Illinois who'll be furious if they read that a Bulgarian defector is being left high and dry in London." Hyland instantly reached for a car phone and called the White House. An hour later he came to me and said, "Your defector will be on a plane tonight." And so he was. He proved to be a cad, dumping Milly's friend as soon as he was safe. But Milly appreciated my effort. And she expected me to learn from the experience how powerful I could be and to act accordingly in the future. It would take a very long time for that lesson to sink in.

I regard one other endeavor as an unqualified success. Months in advance of Milly's fortieth birthday in January 1980, I stole her address book and sent out several dozen invitations to a surprise party for her, marked "Top Secret." She complained for days that the book was missing and was suspicious when it suddenly turned up, but she didn't discover the plot. Among those I invited were her foster sister Lori and several of her neighborhood girlfriends from Chicago, plus her sister Alex, who lives in England. On the day of the party a blizzard unloaded on Washington, but the guests made it into town just before the airport closed. Milly suspected nothing as we arrived at a neighbor's house for what she thought was a small birthday dinner. A deafening roar greeted her when she opened the door and was embraced by some people she hadn't seen in years. The toasts were lavish and loving. I had hired a small band for dancing. Milly was overjoyed at the event. But her memorable comment to me was, "Why, you could have an affair and I'd never know it!" Well, I wouldn't and I couldn't, even had I been inclined toward such a thing. Milly had our children convinced that she always knew what was going on, even if she didn't fully. And she had me convinced, too.

Besides, I was too preoccupied with my career, and I was gradually beginning to make it professionally. I wrote about politics as well as foreign affairs for *The New Republic* and eventually inherited its "White House Watch" column. I wrote a monthly column for the *Wall Street Journal* op-ed page and was a regular commentator on National Public Radio. I started doing commercial radio talk shows and met the former Nixon White House aide and ex–Jesuit priest John McLaughlin, who invited me to join *The McLaughlin Group* when he started his TV show in 1982. The show was a hit, even if widely disparaged for its raucousness. Thanks to it, more officials answered my phone calls, so my print journalism improved. I was a 1984 presidential debate panelist. Then, in 1985, I made the huge mistake of taking the job of Washington bureau chief of *Newsweek*.

Milly was against this move from the beginning. She said she liked *The New Republic*, the things I wrote, and the people, especially Charles Krauthammer, a fellow senior editor, and Michael Kinsley, the editor. She said that *Newsweek* was superficial. She also didn't like it that others had turned down the bureau chief's job and that the New York editors wouldn't let me talk to the Washington staff to ask why. I was too ambitious to listen to her, but she was dead right. The post required a skilled politician, manager, and leader, and I was none of those things. I didn't run the bureau; I let its neuroses and minutiae run me. New York editors and my Washington reporters played political games that I was often oblivious to. Good people were hired away, and I stupidly threw lavish good-bye parties for them, rewarding defection. The post had prestige, though, and suddenly we were invited to the fanciest of dinner parties, especially those at the home of Katharine Graham, publisher of the *Washington Post* and *Newsweek*.

I, of course, was utterly intimidated by Mrs. Graham and found it impossible to connect with her on a human level even though she tried to connect with me. One day beside a tennis court she told Milly and me about the treatment that she and other wives of important Washington males had endured during the 1950s and 1960s. The men, especially those around President Kennedy, she said, were really only interested in girls or other men—for different reasons, of course. Their own wives they tended to patronize or ignore, and the women were expected to put up with it. Milly and I both sat stunned as she recounted details, mumbling that this was horrible. It was one occasion when Milly did not have something penetrating to offer.

In spite of this obvious attempt to establish some rapport, I found it impossible ever to have a relaxed conversation with Mrs. Graham. I took her every request as a royal command. Milly liked Mrs. Graham but simply refused to be at her beck and call. We were regularly asked to be fixtures at her dinners. I always went, but Milly would not, claiming that she had clients to see or that Alex and Andréa—then in their teens—needed her at home.

We fought about that. In fact, we argued constantly for the whole first half of the thirty-three years we've been married. Often it was over Milly's projects. Or the fact that always, always, there were people at our house. Some dropped in for a few hours, some stayed for months. We had a series of au pairs when the kids were little. Milly welcomed in friends who'd left their husbands. One time one of these friends brought her new boyfriend to stay for a month or two. Milly's nephew from Chicago lived with us for two years, supposedly attending college but actually goofing off. When both our girls had left for college, Milly let in a friend of

Andréa's whose parents had kicked her out of the house. With a deep antisocial streak, I wanted solitude, but there wasn't much. I often let visitors know how little I wanted them around. Sometimes I ignored them, speaking to Milly as if they weren't there. Sometimes I made unpleasant faces or groaned when they showed up at our door. Sometimes I demanded to know from Milly how long they would be with us—loudly enough that they could hear. My inhospitality was another thing we fought about.

Milly was also furious, and legitimately, that when I got home from work I had no regard for the fact that she was seeing clients in her office in our basement. Jealous for her attention, I stomped around in the kitchen above and yelled down to her when I couldn't find something. Ultimately she rented an office nearby, across from the girls' high school.

I felt that Milly was forever imposing her people and projects on me, but that I could get nowhere with *my* projects. One of those was religious education for our kids. I was raised as a Presbyterian, but it was important to Milly that the girls be baptized as Catholics. So they were—albeit with the Protestant Mastermans and Jill, who is Jewish, as their godparents. When they were five and six I thought they needed to have some grounding in religion. Roman Catholicism was all right with me, and a friend recommended Holy Trinity in Georgetown, the Kennedy church. I liked it. It had a guitar mass, an eloquent homilist, and a tony congregation.

The enterprise was a disaster, however. It was an eight-mile drive from Chevy Chase to Georgetown, and parking was impossible. So every Sunday I'd try to roust Milly and the girls at 8:30 to get dressed and into the car in time to make 10:30 Mass. I'd yell. I'd implore. But every week we wouldn't leave until 10:15 or 10:20. I'd drive near-recklessly, screaming and swearing at them for their uncooperativeness. There would be no place to park, and it was always standing room only in the church. The next week I'd start yelling earlier and louder, to no avail. An experience that was supposed to be uplifting was becoming semi-traumatic, loaded more with goddammits than with God. After six months I gave up, and the girls—to my continuing regret—got no religious education. Milly now claims that she had no objection to Sunday School for the kids, but that we should have found a church closer to home. I remember no such suggestion at the time, however.

Milly and I fought morning and night, and sometimes by telephone during the day. I'd blame her when the checking account was overdrawn, or for committing me to do something I didn't want to do. She'd blame me for never wanting to do anything or for treating someone badly—in fact, for treating lots of people badly. I'd feel stung and start yelling. When the fight was about one of her projects, I'd often perform a mock military salute, vibrating my hand like a British private in the presence of a general.

Invariably our fight would escalate and raise the issue of power—the fact that she had it and I didn't. She was a gifted arguer, and if she was in danger of losing a point she'd deftly shift to stronger ground. Then I'd raise the stakes. We often fought in bed until two or three in the morning. Losing, I'd desperately escalate, suggest that maybe we should think about getting divorced, then feel desperate and guilty when she said maybe we should. Somehow, within minutes of such discussions, we'd end up apologizing and making love. But in the end she almost always won the argument.

There was never a possibility that we would get divorced. We were committed to each other, bonded, almost welded. Neither of us was ever unfaithful to the other, or even seriously tempted.

We had similar tastes in color, style, and furniture. We were almost telepathic with each other, automatically knowing what the other thought or felt about things. Even though our politics diverged—I stopped being a liberal over foreign policy issues in the late 1970s—we had the same basic values. We mutually adored our children. I respected all her strengths, and she clearly found some in me.

Because of our incessant fighting, we enrolled in marriage counseling and group therapy on various occasions, without much effect. Finally we somehow decided that I would profit from depth therapy, and someone recommended a pricey psychoanalyst. For six years I saw him, three times a week at first. I lay on a couch and talked. He smoked cigars behind me and rarely spoke. All the time and money produced only three conclusions: that I was intensely—and uselessly—envious of my betters in journalism. That I found it almost impossible to recognize, let alone enjoy, the good things that came to me. And that I was deeply resentful toward my wife. The analyst concluded, "The only way you can talk to your wife is on your knees." He said he thought—or thought that I thought—that if I ever stood up on my feet our marriage would end. This idea so disturbed me that I stopped seeing the analyst. Years later we started seeing another therapist, Dr. Dorree Lynn, who'd been a professional mentor to Milly. She began helping us work on our mutual and individual anxieties. More important, she has helped us cope with the mental torment of Parkinson's.

After the fact, Milly has told me that the closest she came to leaving me was over alcohol. Alcoholism runs in my family, and even though I saw alcohol and smoking destroy my father's health—kill him, in fact, at age sixty-three—I did not appreciate that they were threats to me. I started smoking in high school when I got my first newspaper job, but I never drank then. I got drunk in college a few times, no more. I drank martinis as a young reporter in Chicago without ill effects. I began drinking too much in Washington, although at first it caused only trifling embarrassments—wineglasses knocked over on tablecloths or stupid, repetitious political rants at dinner parties—and an occasional near-miss in traffic.

Increasingly, though, I used alcohol to anesthetize myself from the perpetual fear that I lacked the talent to make it in the journalistic big leagues and might even be dismissed from the perch I occupied—as actually happened at *Newsweek*. I assume I also used it to numb my feelings of inferiority at home. And also, excessive drinking simply became a habit. I never drank during the workday. But I would drink a bottle of wine every night during the week. On weekends I would start with very strong gin and tonics about 5:00 P.M. and stay buzzed for the rest of the evening. I would drive drunk to dinner parties and bite my hand to stay awake during the conversation. I would get the hiccups and retreat to the bathroom to put my finger down my throat—and curse at myself in the mirror. I quit smoking when my body told me I had to: my first cigarette in the morning started causing me nearly to faint. But I did not quit drinking even though I would often wake up at 3:00 A.M. and be unable to get back to sleep, then be hung over for much of the next day.

I quit because Milly made me. At first she attacked the symptoms of my alcoholism—my inane dogmatism at dinner tables, the hiccups, my inability to finish helping the kids with homework, and my dangerous driving. Eventually she confronted me with the accusation, "You are an alcoholic." I resented and resisted it. When new evidence arose, as it did almost daily, she bore in, telling me what I was and demanding that I admit it. We began fighting over that. Often, in a rage, she would empty every liquor and wine bottle she could find into a sink. I told her to go ahead; I could always buy more. I also found hiding places for the booze.

Alcohol became the dominant subject of our arguments. Following the usual pattern, the battle ended with Milly's victory. I finally admitted that I was an alcoholic and vowed to do something about it. I consulted the analyst, who said that when my deeper problems were resolved my need for booze would disappear, too. I tried this logic out on Milly, but she guffawed. I kept drinking, and my arguments with Milly worsened. At one stage I got a prescription for Antabuse, a drug that causes violent sickness if mixed with alcohol. That didn't work; I played games with it, calibrating how many days I had to be off it before I could drink again.

Two events triggered her victory. One day in 1986 Milly and I were watching television with our daughter Alex, then a high school senior. A character in a drama used the Spanish word *boracho*—drunk. Alex, who'd many times heard Milly railing about alcohol, pointed to me and said, "Este hombre es un boracho." There was a frozen silence for a second. Then I became outraged, reached for the phone, and made a reservation for myself at a hotel. No one stopped me. I did not leave but made a serious vow to quit.

I didn't do so, though. It took another incident. On the Sunday after Thanksgiving in 1986, we had dinner with a State Department official and a Senate staffer. The next day I called the staffer, who marveled at all the secrets about Reagan administration Central America military and diplomatic strategy that the official had unloaded on us. I had no memory of any of it. That night I attended my first meeting of Alcoholics Anonymous. I have not had a drink since.

This didn't end our arguing, of course. There was always money, visitors, and politics. Of all Milly's many projects, though, her anti-alcohol campaign is one of those about which I am most grateful. It may have saved my life and my marriage. This last exercise of Milly's old power also made it possible for me to cope with, not try to escape from, the challenges ahead. A year and a month from the day I quit drinking, the first signs of Milly's Parkinson's disease appeared.

3

Invasion

For nearly two decades we spent every Christmas vacation in Vermont with Milly's sister Alex, her husband, Paul Wheeler, their daughter and son, and their houseful of guests. Paul, a British film writer, thought that the Bing Crosby movie *Holiday Inn* represented the perfect Christmas. So he and Alex traveled to the United States each year beginning in 1973. The next year, he rented a big house that Jill Schuker found near Windsor, Vermont, filling it with his American friends and some of ours. Later he and Alex bought their own place near Chester, and Christmastime there became a tradition filled with merriment—and conflict.

We skied by day at Bromley, Okemo, or Magic Mountain and gathered for loud, crowded dinners each night. As at our Thanksgivings at home, Milly established the rule that children ate with the adults and took part in conversations. It was also a tradition that on Christmas mornings gifts were opened one at a time so that everyone could appreciate what everyone else had given and received. This rule, combined with the sheer quantity of presents, meant that we started opening at seven, broke for breakfast around nine, and didn't finish until well after lunchtime. I ritually grumbled that the extravagance was obscene, but I was ritually ignored.

Conflict in Vermont mainly had to do with disciplining children. The kids' dorm periodically became a cauldron of rivalry and bullying and, when they got older, a place for experimenting with drugs, alcohol, and sex. When my kids were little and got into fights my impulse was to spank them or sometimes slap them on the head. Milly's practice was to settle quarrels and teach accommodation. Kids who felt hurt or ill-used went running to her for comfort, and she got into disputes with other parents, especially Paul, over how to mete out justice. Milly never hid her opinions. Paul invariably said, "Let 'em handle it themselves." Milly favored supervised negotiation. Also, even though the Wheelers have been lovingly married for nearly forty years, Alex frequently had complaints about Paul that she unburdened upon Milly. And Milly and her sister had their own leftover sibling troubles to resolve. While I made myself useful by cooking meals, washing dishes, and organizing visits from Santa, I used alcohol to make myself as oblivious as possible to the interpersonal goings-on. During our nine-hour drive back to Washington every year, the girls and Milly minutely reviewed the wrongs done over the vacation by various children and adults. Milly also berated me for being inattentive to problems she was trying to solve.

In 1987, the second year I stayed sober and could be of assistance, we decided to alter the tradition by renting a separate house in order to help Andréa with her college applications in peace and quiet. It was there that the first shadow of Parkinson's disease cast itself upon our lives. Milly was writing a check to accompany one of the applications and remarked that she could not form the letter K correctly. She got a piece of paper and wrote her signature four or five more times, then more times, and said her handwriting just wasn't right. I saw no difference. Anyway, I thought Milly was both vain and perfectionist about her clear penmanship. Whatever was wrong—if anything was wrong—was in her imagination or was being exaggerated, I figured.

Over the next five months Milly persisted in saying that her handwriting was changing. Her script was getting smaller, she said, and the flow was losing its smoothness. I finally noticed a change, too, but I assumed it had something to do with the periodic numbness she'd experienced in her hands since early in our marriage, when she'd gotten frostbite in Aspen. I had been determined that Milly learn fashionable skills like skiing and had goaded her into staying out to finish her afternoon lesson even though it was getting cold. Milly also noticed that when she pressed down on the little finger of her right hand it developed a tremor. And she said she felt tingling in her hands.

In May, Milly made an appointment to see her old boss at the Neurology Center in Bethesda, Maryland, Dr. Marvin Korengold. For a few years after earning her master's degree she had worked there counseling patients with chronic illnesses and their families. It was hard work. The diseases the patients suffered from—multiple sclerosis, Alzheimer's, amyotrophic lateral sclerosis (ALS, or Lou Gehrig's disease), epilepsy—were often devastating and incurable, and Milly occasionally brought home harrowing stories of families torn apart by the burden. She was particularly shaken over the case of a woman stricken with guilt because she'd left her father, a Parkinson's victim, at home by himself. He fell and lay on the floor unable to rise for half a day, with no one there to help him. This story triggered something deep in Milly, perhaps guilt at being unable to help her own father after he suffered his stroke, perhaps empathy with the father's dependency. Physical illness was one of the few things in life that scared Milly. It was always a byword with her that "as long as you've got your health, you can handle everything else." Whenever she prayed, it was for health for herself and our family.

Dr. Korengold examined Milly and diagnosed ulnar neuropathy, a nerve inflamed from pressure at the elbow. He told her to try to keep her arms straight and avoid leaning on the elbow. Milly reported these findings to me with relief that the problem was not serious. But even though she followed instructions, her symptoms did not go away. On a follow-up visit in June, Korengold's records show, he had her swing her arms and noticed that the right did not move as smoothly as the left. He prescribed Symmetrel, which Milly took believing it was meant to help her nerve problem. He did not tell her what it was actually for, evidently not wanting to scare her. She went back to see Korengold a few times during the summer because her right little finger remained weak and she began to notice a slight tremor in her right foot when she pressed the accelerator or brake while driving.

One day in September she called me at work in tears, with a panic in her voice that I'd never heard before. "Something terrible has happened," she said. "You've got to come home." I had a fleeting terror that one of the girls had been injured or killed. She said, "I looked up the medicine Korengold gave me in my pill book. Symmetrel is for Parkinson's disease!" I was relieved that this was not the worst possible news, but for Milly it was. "I know what Parkinson's is. I've seen people with it," she cried. "It's a horrible disease. People shake. They can't walk. They choke on their food. It can't be that!" She said she had torn up Korengold's prescription, thrown away the medicine she had, and would never speak to him again.

I drove home as soon as I could and found Milly utterly distraught. She paced around our bedroom, showed me the medicine and prescription in the wastebasket, repeated what she'd told me on the phone, and said she hated Korengold. She also recalled the story of the man who'd fallen and was unable to rise. She said she would end up just like him. This was the first time in our lives together that I had ever seen Milly out of control. She said that if she did have Parkinson's it meant that she would have to give up her practice because clients would not want to be treated by someone "so pathetic." She predicted, "You won't keep loving me. You'll leave me."

I hugged her and told her that this would never happen. In the moment, I said it mainly to ease her distress and the confusion it caused me. Seeing Milly so upset scared me. But I also meant what I said completely. I could not imagine anything that could ever cause me to leave Milly or stop loving her.

She read my mind. "You don't know what Parkinson's does to people. You'll have to take me to the bathroom. You'll have to feed me. You won't want to do that," she said.

I said rather automatically that I didn't care what happened, I'd never leave her. I meant this, too, although she was correct: I knew nothing about Parkinson's or the extreme disabilities it could cause. And, of course, her problems then were so mild that her grim predictions seemed speculative and extreme.

I tried another tack that did ease her anxiety. "Look, we don't even know that you really have Parkinson's. A couple of months ago it was ulnar neuropathy. We've got to check this out. You're assuming the worst before you know what's going on."

In spite of her vow never to see Dr. Korengold again, she went back a few days later, and I went with her. Milly had been a popular employee at the Neurology Center, and because she was clearly distraught about his tentative diagnosis, Korengold asked some of his colleagues to help examine her. This was the first neurological exam I witnessed; Milly has now undergone hundreds of them in various doctors' offices. Korengold had her stretch out her arms and try to hold her hands steady. Then he asked her to quickly tap the thumb and index finger of each hand. After that, to touch one index finger to her nose, then the other. Next, to flop her hands, palms up and down. He told her to look at his finger and follow it with her eyes. He asked her to blink, then wink one eye and then the other. He had her tap the toes of one foot and then the other. He hit her knees with a rubber hammer. He asked her to walk down a hallway, swinging her arms. Finally he had her sit down and write some sentences on a piece of paper.

Milly acted as though she were being interrogated by the Inquisition. With each task, she looked nervously at the doctors for signs of whether she was passing or failing, with failure meaning that she might be doomed. The doctors tried to calm her fears, but by the end it seemed to me she was quaking as much in fright as from any neurological problem. Before passing judgment, Korengold huddled with his colleagues, leaving Milly and me alone in an examining room. Milly was weeping, sure that Korengold was going to condemn her with his diagnosis. I tried to tell her that I hadn't seen anything to be alarmed about. I did not tell her that I had noticed that the movements of her left hand were slightly quicker and more facile than those on the right. I also said that, whatever the verdict was here, we would get a second opinion elsewhere.

Korengold returned and apologetically said that he and his colleagues were pretty sure that the tiny impairments on her right side were evidence of Parkinson's. Milly again started to cry, clearly disconcerting Korengold. He tried to reassure us by saying that trajectories for people with Parkinson's vary widely and that some people's symptoms remain mild for years. He cited the case of a dentist who was still practicing and playing golf twenty years after being diagnosed. And, he said, so much promising research work was being done on Parkinson's that a cure might be found within a decade. He gave us some literature on Parkinson's and suggested that we join a support group for patients and their families.

Milly cried and her body shook as we left the building to go to our car. I held her close around the shoulders and tried to be consoling, assuring her that this diagnosis was not necessarily final. When she stopped crying, she said that she would never see Korengold again. She vowed anew that she would not take the medicine he had prescribed. And she said she would never attend a support group. Seeing people with advanced Parkinson's would make her more depressed than she already was, she said.

We began a lengthy process of diagnosis-shopping. Milly was desperate to find someone who would tell her that she did not have Parkinson's. I, too, fervently hoped that something like Korengold's first diagnosis would prove correct, though mainly because I wanted to restore Milly's peace of mind and the serenity of our household. Since I knew so little about Parkinson's, I had only the vaguest sense that Milly's life and both of our futures hung in the balance. I simply knew that we had to find out what the truth was because the possibility of Parkinson's was so unsettling to Milly. So we immediately set about looking for places to go for a second opinion.

In the meantime I also started researching Parkinson's. The disease is named for the British physician James Parkinson, who wrote the first scholarly paper on the "shaking palsy" in 1812. As always, I was inclined to accept expert opinion, and I allowed

Korengold's optimism to dominate my thinking and my words to Milly. Each time she told me how she feared being incapacitated, I reminded her of Korengold's golf-playing dentist. In the literature I read on Parkinson's, however, I could not escape the menacing words "degenerative . . . incurable . . . progressively disabling . . . sometimes fatal." I saw these words, but I could not absorb them emotionally and simply refused to accept them as a prediction for Milly. I comforted myself with the assurances in the literature that "medication can alleviate symptoms and improve quality of life for many years" and with the long list of experimental therapies promising to bring the disease under control. The literature said, encouragingly, that Parkinson's was primarily a disease of the aged—Milly was just forty-eight at the time—but it also reported that the average age of onset was descending, for reasons no one could explain. Whenever Milly saw me looking at a Parkinson's article and asked me what it said, I would read aloud the material that gave reasons for hope and skip what I feared would heighten her distress.

Even though Milly rejected Korengold's diagnosis, she was haunted by it. She took it as a curse. She could talk about little else. She told me she was convinced that she would be abandoned—as she was by her mother, and as her father was by many of his labor union friends when he was disabled and being pursued by the government. Milly's foster mother told me later that, as a little child, Milly cried whenever her dress got soiled and tried to cover up the stains with her hands. Evidently she feared she would be rejected if she were dirty. Now she seemed terrified that her hands would shake and she would not be able to hide them.

With some of her friends and co-therapists—even more than with me, at least then—she wept uncontrollably and said she was sure that I would find her "disgusting" and leave her. She said she had known several patients at the Neurology Center whose husbands promised to stand by them when they got sick but ultimately didn't. Judy Siegel, our neighbor, says that Milly sometimes seemed interested in reports about people who were successfully coping with Parkinson's. At other times, though, she could talk only about the "horrible" condition she expected to be in and predicted that I would find another woman, leaving her to deteriorate alone.

Similarly, Jill Schuker remembers Milly being totally consumed by the diagnosis and determined to prove it wrong. After years of long, lighthearted shopping trips with Milly and endless discussions about our kids and her career and love life, Jill suddenly found Milly able to talk about one thing only. Milly irrationally demanded that Jill save her from Parkinson's. "Figure out a cure," she cried. "You can do it!" Even though Milly was normally protective of Andréa, she was so upset that she burdened Andréa with her fears of being left by me. Andréa had seen the fathers of two of her close friends leave when their wives got sick and thought it was a possibility that this might happen to us. She worried that she might end up as Milly's caretaker.

I can understand why Milly and Andréa might have worried. There had been mercifully little illness in our family, but when there was I did not deal with it well. I was a bystander as Milly did most of the work to cope with Andréa's dyslexia. Later I was at first dismissive and then struck an "Oh God, what now?" attitude when Milly became concerned that Andréa was gaining weight and becoming uncharacteristically lethargic in high school. It was Milly who took her from specialist to specialist until someone diagnosed hypothyroidism and prescribed corrective medicine. When Milly went to the hospital for surgical removal of hemorrhoids, I was attentive until she had been back home for a few days. When she complained constantly about pain, didn't want to get out of bed, and had to be helped to the bathroom, I did what needed doing, but I made my impatience clear and even accused her of whining. I acted as though shaming would hasten her recovery. I showed no tolerance for her dependency. In the traumatic aftermath of Korengold's diagnosis, I was comforting and attentive. But on the basis of her experience with me after her surgery, there was good reason for Milly to fear that I would be unsupportive, or even nasty, under the pressure of a long, debilitating illness.

In the meantime, some of Milly's friends thought that she was overreacting to her symptoms and the tentative diagnosis. In fact, a few of them have told me they doubted that she really had a physical problem and wondered whether she was suffering from hypochondria or some psychosomatic hysteria. They thought her symptoms might be related to menopause, or to our daughter Alex's departure for college and Andréa's preparations to go. Milly's distress was great enough, though, that a psychiatrist friend prescribed Valium for anxiety and Desyrel for depression. These helped only modestly.

In November 1988, we went to Johns Hopkins University in Baltimore to see Dr. Mahlon DeLong, who later became Milly's regular neurologist. DeLong is a gentle, scholarly man with a high-domed bald head and thick glasses. Milly broke down and sobbed as she told him about Korengold's diagnosis, what she had seen of Parkinson's, and what she feared for herself. He calmed her and then conducted the same basic exam as Korengold's. To our huge relief, DeLong said that her symptoms were too indistinct for him to make any definite diagnosis. He said he thought that depression and anxiety were her dominant problems and suggested that she see a psychotherapist.

She did that and in January 1989 also consulted an orthope-
dist, who said he was certain that she had serious ulnar neuropathy. He added that she might also be suffering from thoracic
outlet syndrome, a pinching of a nerve as it passes through the
shoulder area. He sent her to a physical therapist, who gave her
an exercise regimen. Someone also gave her the name of a surgeon in Boston to consult if her symptoms persisted. The revived
diagnosis of neuropathy was like a stay of execution for Milly. It
created great hope that both of us clung to and pretended to believe in. But we both knew that *this* diagnosis might be wrong.
Milly dutifully did her hand-strength exercises, but they seemed
to have no effect on her symptoms.

I decided that we should get definitive answers to Milly's
problems by having her undergo a complete physical at the Mayo
Clinic in Rochester, Minnesota. We went in early April, in both
hope and trepidation, holding hands constantly. We spent three
days there. During the first two, Milly underwent blood tests,
nerve conduction studies, and x-rays of her spine, shoulder, and
elbows. I trailed her, trying to keep her spirits up between tests,
but mostly reading magazines in waiting rooms. The crucial neurological exam was scheduled for the third day.

On the way to the clinic that chilly, cloudy morning we
stopped at a church. Always a believer in God, I had become
more religious through AA and had begun attending an Episcopal
church in Washington. The Rochester church was Lutheran, an
imposing brick building with a dim interior. We knelt, and I fervently asked God please to let Milly not be diagnosed with
Parkinson's disease. We left a contribution and picked up small sil-
very lapel crosses that we have to this day.

An hour later our prayers seemed to be answered. Mayo's neurologist was a kindly older man with a Hispanic name, which

Milly took as a good omen. She told him that she had been diagnosed with both ulnar neuropathy and Parkinson's and tearfully said she was terrified at the prospect of Parkinson's. She made it plain that she was desperate that he not discover Parkinson's. I had a flash of worry that she might bias his judgment. But then I figured that this was the Mayo Clinic, one of the best medical facilities in the world, and that sympathy wouldn't overcome science.

The doctor gave her the usual exam. There was a tremor in Milly's little finger when she held out her arm, but it went away when she rested her hand on his exam table. He said, "Do you see that? That means you don't have Parkinson's. You have what's called essential tremor. Lots of people have it. It's benign. It won't get any worse. The nice thing is, you can help control it with a glass of wine at dinner. And the x-rays show you don't have ulnar neuropathy or thoracic outlet syndrome either."

We returned home filled with relief and joy. But it was short-lived. Milly soon noticed that she was losing strength in her right hand—especially, she said, when she was washing her hair. She said she could not hold a pencil correctly or use tweezers. And there *was* a tremor in her little finger when her hand was at rest. Milly became agitated and depressed again. She got her internist and a psychiatrist to give her prescriptions for Valium, Prozac for depression, and also Xanax, an anti-anxiety drug. And still determined to escape the conclusion that she had Parkinson's, Milly went to Boston with Jill and consulted the orthopedic surgeon who'd been recommended to her. He said he thought she had thoracic outlet syndrome and tentatively scheduled shoulder surgery for July.

Before she underwent an operation, I said, we needed to be sure about what was wrong. I scheduled a return trip to Mayo for late June. This time, in addition to other tests, she had an MRI of the head and spine and a spinal fluid test. The Hispanic doctor had retired—a sign of incompetence, I feared—and she saw a new neurologist. After the customary exam he said that he detected "parkinsonism," but added that the only way to know for certain was for Milly to take Sinemet, or levodopa, the standard drug for Parkinson's. If her symptoms improved—especially if the tremor went away—it would mean she had the disease. This time we left Mayo deeply depressed, but still clinging to hope that L-dopa might not work.

Alas, L-dopa did work. Developed in the 1960s, the drug replaces the dopamine normally produced by a cluster of black cells deep in the brain known collectively as the substantia nigra. Parkinson's symptoms begin to appear when about 70 percent of these cells have died. The cause of their death—or self-destruction, as scientists now describe it—is unknown. Sinemet does not affect cell death, but for several years it adequately provides the dopamine the body needs for fluid motion. Over time, however, it ceases to be as effective, and patients again experience tremor and rigidity, which gradually worsen. Some neurologists believe that prolonged use of L-dopa causes damage to brain circuits, inducing dementia in some patients. It definitely causes hallucinations in others, and sometimes wild gyrations of the neck and arms called dyskinesia. In the true story dramatized in the movie *Awakenings*, L-dopa brought patients out of a mysterious coma, but their dyskinesias were so violent that they chose to return to sleep.

Milly's tremor subsided, and strength returned to her hand. Her handwriting improved. Through this wracking, months-long ordeal, Milly continued her work schedule, seeing clients individually and in group therapy. She kept her office in Bethesda, a few blocks from our home, and also drove to Georgetown two nights a week to lead groups. She remained a strong, involved mother, calling the girls at college almost daily. When she could not reach one of them for a day or two, she would call—or tell me to call—campus security at Dartmouth or Boston College and have the police knock on her dorm door with a message to call home. The girls protested that this was invasive and embarrassing, but they also understood that it was typical of their mom. In her sophomore year at Dartmouth, when Alex became stressed out from overwork, Milly was constantly on the phone with her and ordered her to quit a part-time job she'd taken. Andréa, in her first year at BC, also was homesick and depressed. Once Milly insisted that we fly to Boston to make sure she was okay.

Milly functioned, but the life we had known before her diagnosis was over. Friends still came to call, but they weren't invited to stay over. Parkinson's disease had moved in, invading our home. It was a malevolent presence that became the preoccupation of our lives, crowding everything except our love for each other and for our kids. The definite diagnosis shattered Milly psychologically. She often clung to me and sobbed piteously, sometimes several times a day, saying that her life would be terrible. "Why is God punishing me?" she cried. "I've always tried to be good. What did I do that was bad?"

On occasion she said she had thought that her adulthood would be safe because she had suffered so many losses in childhood. Now, she realized, this was not true. Other times she said she believed she was the latest victim of some family curse. Her mother was mentally unstable. Her father had died young. Her half-brother had suffered from schizophrenia and committed suicide. She told me she was afraid that her clients would find out that she had Parkinson's and leave her practice. Alternatively, she said she was not serving them well because she was so preoccupied with her condition. She also insisted, again and again, that eventually I would stop loving her. "Someday I'm going to kill myself," she said.

I did my best to be reassuring. I told her that she was a great therapist, that she'd helped so many people and was still doing so, that they would not abandon her. I told her she had great friends who loved her. She'd given them so much, I said, that they'd always be there for her. "Your kids love you, and I love you," I said. "No matter what happens, I'm here."

I meant this, utterly. I felt as bonded to Milly as ever. I still adored her smell, taste, and touch. Despite her despair about the future, she remained the Old Milly, decisive about people, politics, and projects. I still yelled when she bounced a check or committed us to see friends of hers when I wanted to vegetate. But we stopped fighting incessantly because our disagreements had lost the power stakes I once had assigned to them. With a twinge of self-importance, I felt as though Milly now needed me more than I needed her for the first time in our marriage. When I agreed to some project of hers—for instance, lending money to our cleaning lady and co-signing a mortgage so that she could buy a townhouse—it seemed like I was participating in a good idea, not caving in to pressure. I felt as though I was no longer her assistant, but her partner.

Despite my attempts at reassurance, Milly often was inconsolable. But Xanax helped. I admit, I was so unsettled by her despair that almost every time she wept I encouraged her to take a pill, which seemed to calm her. She became dependent and took too much of it. She also was taking a dangerous cocktail of other medicines: Sinemet, prescribed in too-large doses by a neurologist we visited in Philadelphia; a Sinemet-booster called Eldepryl;

Prozac; Halcion, a sleeping pill she got through a psychiatrist friend; and an occasional Valium.

Milly lost weight. She had trouble sleeping. And most frighteningly, she often felt faint. The combination of medicines evidently was causing dehydration and depressing her blood pressure. I bought a drugstore blood pressure device and was alarmed by the wild fluctuations it registered. We had to find a doctor close to home, but Milly repeated that she would never see Dr. Korengold again, holding him somehow responsible for her illness. In January 1990, we went back to see Dr. DeLong at Johns Hopkins. He was appalled at the list of drugs she was taking—the combination of Eldepryl and Prozac can be fatal—and set out a regimen for weaning her down. His nurse intervened to suggest that he admit Milly to the hospital, and he agreed that would be the best way to rehydrate her body, begin easing her off Xanax, and lower her dosage of Sinemet.

Her blood pressure returned to normal, and the danger of fainting abated. But then other symptoms developed. For a time, the worst was severe nightly leg cramps. For years Milly and I have closed out our day watching the eleven o'clock local news and then ABC's *Nightline* in bed. But during this period, when Milly tried to get to sleep afterward the muscles in her calves would freeze into tight knots and sometimes jolt with excruciating spasms. I regularly stayed up until two or two-thirty with my head under the covers, rubbing first one leg and then the other. Eventually I had to go to sleep in order to function at work the next day. Then Milly would get up, wandering the house until nearly dawn to make the cramps go away. She was exhausted most of the time and looked emaciated.

She also developed severe upward curling of the toes on her right foot, called dystonia, and the beginnings of slurred speech.

When she swung her arms in an arc, there were hitches in her movement, known as "cogwheeling." These are common symptoms of Parkinson's, especially as Sinemet begins losing its power to fully replace the missing dopamine. In addition, Milly suffered severe back pain that we assumed was related to Parkinson's. Acupuncture and physical therapy did no good, so we went to see a neurosurgeon, who diagnosed a herniated disc. Milly underwent back surgery.

One day in late 1990, Dr. DeLong informed us that he was leaving Hopkins to become chairman of the Neurology Department at Emory University in Atlanta. This was a blow to both of us because up to that point DeLong was the ablest and most empathetic doctor we'd found. But, he said, Emory would give him significant support for the experiments he was doing on monkeys, inducing Parkinson's symptoms chemically and then surgically lancing deep-brain organs to correct the symptoms. At the time I paid little attention to what he said about his research, though it was gaining national attention in scientific journals, because the benefits seemed too distant to have any meaning for Milly. Five years later, though, Milly had one such operation under DeLong's supervision. And three years after that, another.

Besides looking for another neurologist, we searched for other remedies. Milly's foster mother, Annie, believed profoundly in Chinese herbal medicine, as did other members of the Villarreal family. Milly's foster brother, Larry, said he had been cured of severe back pain, and Milly's foster sister, Lori, had been cured of chronic stomach pain. So, on a visit to Chicago, we went to Chinatown, where an herbal doctor held Milly's hand for a moment, said he understood what her problem was, and began reaching into various boxes to assemble what looked like a collection of twigs and tree barks. He also supplied detailed instructions on how to prepare an herbal brew. For months I meticulously followed the directions—boiling, cooling, and reboiling the mixture until it produced an evil-smelling black tea that Milly could barely swallow. Nevertheless, she bravely made herself do so, but without any effect on her symptoms.

Another course was recommended by Milly's friend Gloria Doyle, a former researcher at the *Los Angeles Times* who has a tumor growing on her spinal cord. Surgeons trying to remove the tumor damaged the cord, causing partial paralysis of her legs, and the tumor's continued growth is progressively robbing her of other motor functions. A fighter like Milly, Gloria applied her research skills to the world of alternative medicine and found, among other things, "prano therapy," whose practitioners are licensed in Europe and elsewhere. Gloria and her husband Denis visited one therapist in Milan, Gabriella Passoni, and reported some improvement in feeling in her limbs. She told us that Gabriella was eminent enough that she had spent time at a paralysis center in Florida where her skills were taken seriously. Milly was desperate to try this, and though I doubted it would work for Parkinson's, I couldn't refuse her anything.

So we flew to Italy and visited Gabriella in her basement office for four mornings. A deeply religious woman, Gabriella was convinced that her healing gifts were akin to those of Jesus, but obviously far less powerful. Without question, an unusual heat emanated from her hands. She showed us a sheet of x-ray film with handprints on them that her energy had produced. She also said that part of prano-therapy training in Italy consisted of holding and gently manipulating an orange until it dried out inside. She showed us her petrified orange.

Her therapy consisted partly of massage and partly of flicking her hands over Milly's head, back, and legs "wicking away" "undesirable" energy. Her hands did crackle, and Milly said she felt better after the sessions. We had a delightful mini-vacation in Italy, driving to Lake Como and Venice. But it was clear, as I had feared, that Gabriella's therapy made no lasting impact on Milly's condition. Milly and Gloria read books about alternative therapy, and I heard enough from them that I'm convinced prano therapy merits scientific attention, but Milly's visits to other prano practitioners in the United States did no more good than the one in Italy.

Following a fad made respectable in upscale circles by the journalist Bill Moyers, we also experimented with various mind-body health nostrums. We got audiotapes from some of the country's noted healers and meditation experts and listened to them in bed. Following someone's advice, I tried visualization therapy, calling on Milly to imagine a warm, golden light descending from God, penetrating her brain and restoring life to her dying dopamine cells. None of this had any effect, though Milly did get some mental relief from yoga classes.

We never considered alternative cures a substitute for conventional medicine. And after Dr. DeLong departed for Atlanta, we had to find Milly a new neurologist. She saw several but couldn't find one with whom she shared the chemistry she'd had with De-Long. In late 1991, a friend of Milly's, Sharon Jayne, suggested that we visit her boss, Dr. David Kessler, head of the U.S. Food and Drug Administration, who liked to interview patients as a way of staying in touch with practical medicine. Later famous for his war on tobacco, Kessler asked Milly whether she was willing to become a subject in experimental studies. She said she would do anything that might work, so Kessler said he would call the National Institutes of Health to see whether doctors there would see her.

Milly has been a patient at NIH ever since. The doctors and nurses of the experimental therapeutics branch of the National Institute of Neurological Disorders and Stroke (NINDS) have been Milly's support system for nearly a decade. The chief of that branch, Dr. Tom Chase, now sixty-eight, is a slender, white-haired, career NIH scientist and administrator who has worked with at least two Nobel Prize winners and helped design clinical drug trials that perfected Sinemet and its timed-release variation, Sinemet CR. Over the years Milly has volunteered for a few drug trials, which usually did not produce any beneficial results and sometimes made her feel sick. In terms of medical attention and kindness, however, she and I have received far more than we have given. The nurses, especially Marge Gillespie, compassionately listened to Milly as, visit after visit, she unburdened her despair, many times saying that she intended to commit suicide someday.

Medically all that NIH could do for several years was modulate the basic Parkinson's drugs Milly took, especially Sinemet. In May 1995, one Sinemet experiment led to one of the most harrowing experiences that Milly—and I—have endured during her Parkinson's affliction.

Milly's principal doctor at NIH, Leo Verhagen, began to suspect that she did not have a classic case of Parkinson's because her symptoms did not respond well to Sinemet. He suggested that she enter the hospital, be gradually taken completely off Sinemet, and then receive precisely measured intravenous doses to gauge her response. Perhaps, he said, this would enable him to calculate her ideal dosage.

This procedure proved to be a descent into hell. After a few days without medicine, Milly was totally unable to move, speak, or swallow. She had to be fed intravenously. I watched my wife turn almost into a living corpse, able only to move her eyes, which had a look of terror in them. She could understand what I said when I talked to her, but she could not respond or even squeeze my hand as I held hers.

I appealed to Verhagen to begin giving her Sinemet again, and he agreed that it was time. Over the course of a week she gradually ascended out of hell, but she never regained as much body control as she had before the experiment. Verhagen said the test—lasting twelve days in all—confirmed that her "parkinsonism" consisted of more than simple loss of dopamine. This is not unheard of. About one-third of Parkinson's victims have something vaguely known as "Parkinson's-plus." Milly evidently has it, but no one knows exactly what it is, what causes it, or how to treat it. Various complications of Parkinson's have been identified—multi-system atrophy, Lewy body disease, corticobasal degeneration—but none exactly fits her symptoms. Dr. DeLong later told me that he thought her case sui generis—"Milly Syndrome," he called it.

One definite Parkinson's-plus symptom—and the most dangerous to Milly—is loss of balance. Milly had never been an athlete. No matter how many skiing lessons she took, she stayed on beginner slopes. When we went bike riding she often fell. My reaction, when she was in danger of injury, was to get angry and accuse her of not being careful. And this is how I began to react to her falls. The first serious one was on Saint Martin, the Caribbean island, which we visited on a Christmas–New Year's ocean cruise in 1993 with Milly's foster sister Lori and our families.

I was in a store when one of our daughters ran up to say, "Mom has fallen. Come quick!" Milly had stumbled over a curb and fallen headlong into a street. She had smashed her upper lip and was bleeding badly inside her mouth. My instant reaction was, "Oh, goddammit, Milly. Why can't you be more careful!" But I swallowed the fright and anger, apologized profusely, and got her back to the ship, where the doctor put several stitches in her lip.

It was a pattern that would be repeated over and over. Once we spent a weekend at a friend's home on Nantucket. Milly stumbled at the airport and bruised her lip. Later, at our friend's home, she was sitting on the edge of our bed. Suddenly she keeled over and hit her forehead on the nightstand. We rushed to the hospital for stitches. Another time we were visiting Lori and Jerry Long at their vacation house in Wisconsin. Milly tripped on a rug and fell forward, again hitting her lip and requiring stitches.

The falls were utterly unpredictable and frightening. Milly could go for days without an incident, then fall twice in one day. When she fell, she seemed to have no reflexive ability to put out her arms to break the impact. We became regular visitors to the emergency room at Suburban Hospital near our home. At various times Milly got stitches there in her lips, forehead, chin, and eyebrows. On an early visit I was asked to leave the examining room while the nurse talked to Milly. Clearly she was inquiring about spousal abuse. Later the doctors and nurses regarded our visits as grimly routine. Sometimes I would arrive home when Milly should have been there and chase around looking for signs that she had gone to the hospital. Several times I found a smudge of blood on a bathroom floor or on a rug and drove to the emergency room to find her. NIH assigned Milly to see a physical therapist to teach her how to break her falls, but that did not seem to work. I bought her a kayaking helmet, but she refused to wear it.

Ultimately she needed a walker. For a while we were constantly trying new models—with wheels, without wheels, with and without handbrakes. Some worked for a time, but eventually she fell despite the walker—or on top of it, causing another injury. She was determined to stay out of a wheelchair. Milly insisted on walking and also driving her car. Her office garage had terribly narrow parking spaces, and her car gradually began to look like the loser in a demolition derby. Milly's face intermittently was a mass of scars and bruises. She often said, "Look at how ugly I am." I'd reply, "You look like you have been through a prize fight, but you are still beautiful."

Milly stopped driving in 1994 after she bumped into the rear of another car at a stop sign. Evidently her foot slipped from the brake as she was slowing down. She didn't hit the other car hard or do any damage. But the driver, a huge man, jumped out and demanded to see her license and registration. He identified himself as a lawyer—he turned out to be a mere paralegal—and accused Milly, whose medicine was not working, of being drunk. He called the police on a cell phone. They arrived, interviewed everyone, and, of course, declined to press charges. But Milly was so shaken by the experience that she started taking cabs or getting rides to work and eventually decided to move her office back to our basement. But that magnified the risk—all too imminent—of her falling down stairs.

One day in October 1995, I pulled onto our block and found fire trucks and an ambulance on the street. A neighbor said, "They're at your house." I ran up to find Milly inside the ambulance, being comforted by her sister Alex, who had been visiting from England. Milly was on a stretcher, her neck in a brace. Alex said she thought Milly was not badly injured, though she was going to the hospital for x-rays. Alex said she had been cooking and heard Milly scream and fall—backward, as it turned out—down a full flight of stairs. Alex said she'd rushed to help and left the pan on the stove, which burned and scorched the kitchen ceiling.

It was a miracle that Milly was unhurt, but this accident terrified us both. It conjured up the worst case of Parkinson's we knew about—that of the onetime Democratic presidential candidate and congressman Morris Udall, who had fallen down stairs a few years earlier and thereafter was confined to a hospital room, unable to move, eat, or talk and had to be fed through a feeding tube. We had lived in our beloved Chevy Chase home for nearly twenty years when this fall occurred, but I knew that we would soon have to leave.

Loss of balance was Milly's most menacing symptom, but it was not the only one. Like many other Parkinson's victims, she gradually became unable to voluntarily turn in bed. On the other hand, she was also in danger of sliding out of bed at night, and we had to install a partial railing both to keep her in and give her something to hold on to when she was sitting on the edge. She complained more than anything else about a persistent pursing, or dystonia, of her lips that she said made her feel sick. Periodically, when her Sinemet unaccountably "turned off," she also became frozen in a chair, unable to move her arms or legs. On one occasion, we were at a dinner party and when it was time to move from the living room to the table Milly could not lift herself. She had a stunned, frightened expression on her face. After several minutes the paralysis passed, and she made it to the table. Milly also reported that several times she had been frozen while doing therapy.

As Milly's condition got worse, we began looking at drastic surgical therapies to relieve the symptoms. Basically, two were available—a fetal cell transplant and a pallidotomy. I read a lot about both. In 1994 Milly and I had met up with Joan Samuelson, president of the Parkinson's Action Network, who got us involved in advocacy and lobbying for increased federal funding of Parkinson's research. Joan put us in touch with some of the top neurologists in the country, whom I called for advice about what we should do next for Milly.

They told me that, theoretically, a fetal transplant would be the most advisable thing to do for a direct hit at Milly's Parkinson's. The procedure, made controversial by opposition from the right-to-life movement, involves injecting dopamine-producing cells from aborted fetuses into the brain of a Parkinson's victim to replace those that have died. At the time we were considering the operation, federally sponsored research trials were just beginning because a ban imposed by the Reagan and Bush administrations had only recently been lifted.

A few doctors were performing the operation without federal sponsorship, notably a surgeon in California who was reporting dramatic results and had been featured on a national TV magazine show. But the researchers I talked to warned me away from him, saying that he was not publishing any scholarly findings and stories were circulating about botched operations and brain damage. When he was unable to obtain enough aborted fetuses in the United States, the critics said, this doctor would take a patient to Japan. He'd open a hole in the patient's head there, then fly the patient to China, where aborted fetal tissue is easily obtainable—it takes material from about seven fetuses for each implant—and complete the procedure. I'd heard that Chinese hospitals were filthy. I was not about to trust this guy with Milly.

The experts I consulted also said that their review of results from Europe and elsewhere indicated that while fetal transplantation was a promising area of research, there were significant problems keeping cells alive after they were transferred. They advised looking seriously into pallidotomy instead.

This was the operation Dr. DeLong had been studying. Because of him, Milly decided that she wanted it. And she wanted him to do it. We hadn't seen DeLong in more than four years, but he was happy to hear from us again and gave us an appointment in September 1995 for a consultation. We flew to Atlanta in trepidation, fearful that DeLong might not think Milly was a good candidate for a pallidotomy. It was reassuring that he hadn't changed much. He was still gentle and soft-spoken. He was just getting balder. He gave Milly the usual exam, noting that her condition had become a lot worse since he'd last seen her. Then, to our relief and delight, he said he thought that pallidotomy might work for her.

He explained the procedure. It was a daylong operation in which Milly would be awake throughout, helping to guide doctors to the targets they would be trying to hit deep in her brain. First they would insert a long, fine probe to electronically "map" the globus pallidus, a centimeter-long neurological "circuit box," to find the exact places affecting movement of her arms, fingers, legs, and face. Once the mapping was completed, another probe would be inserted to singe the organ at the correct spots.

Mahlon DeLong was fifty-seven at this time. A Californian whose father had been a gold prospector and town clerk, DeLong had gone to Stanford, where he fell in love with scientific research. He did not decide to be a physician until his senior year, but he still got into Harvard Medical School, where he became interested in neuroscience, then a new field. Before moving to Johns Hopkins, he spent five years at the National Institute of Mental Health, part of the National Institutes of Health in

Bethesda, doing research on techniques for recording the activity of brain cells.

He'd been interested from the outset in Parkinson's and the organs involved in it, located in a deep-brain region called the basal ganglia. In 1990, the year he treated Milly, he published the findings that established his eminence. His research on monkeys showed that Parkinson's symptoms—especially tremor and stiffness—don't result from diminished activity in the circuits of the basal ganglia, but from hyperactivity in the subthalamic nucleus (STN), a kind of internal regulator for brain signals. This excess STN activity translates into excessive braking of mobility by a nearby structure, the globus pallidus. He showed that the symptoms could be reduced by doing microscopic damage to the STN. At first he was worried, though, that inflicting lesions in the STN in humans might cause unwelcome complications, so he began experimenting on the globus pallidus. He'd begun doing pallidotomies on people in 1992.

DeLong said—and I had read in various articles—that some patients experienced dramatic improvement from the operation. He cautioned that others showed little improvement, though. And both he and the literature warned that there was potential danger. Some patients suffered brain hemorrhages. Others, because the globus pallidus sits immediately atop the optic nerve, were rendered permanently blind by a surgical accident. None of this had happened at Emory, he said, but we had to take the risk into account.

Milly dismissed the danger and begged him to perform the surgery. "I can't stand to live this way anymore," she said. "I'd rather die."

He agreed to do it.

4

Heroine

A hospital attendant stuck her head into the waiting room and chirped, "Would you like to wish good luck to the patient?" We leapt out of our seats and into the hallway. Our daughter Alex, first out of the door, took one look at Milly and burst into tears.

Milly was being rolled out of a prep room in a wheelchair toward an elevator. Her head was surrounded by a square, gold-colored metal frame that looked like an instrument of medieval torture. It's called a "halo" and serves the godly purpose of healing. But it looks obscene. It was screwed to Milly's skull in four places. We could not see the two pins at the back of her head, but the two in front were obviously penetrating the skin and flesh of her forehead, which was pinched and rust-colored from disinfectant.

It was quickly clear that Milly was not suffering any pain from the penetration. Characteristically, she immediately asked us how she looked. I told her she appeared ready for transport into some other dimension. She'd been given a local anesthetic where the halo was attached and was mildly sedated to keep her calm for a CAT scan and the early phases of surgery. However, Andréa did not know this when she ran up to join us at the elevator door—I don't know where she'd been—and when she saw Milly, she burst into tears, too.

We rode on the elevator with her—me, Alex, Andréa, Milly's foster sister Lori, Joan Samuelson of the Parkinson's Action Network, and our goddaughter, Jenny Cabrera. The girls and I kissed Milly through the contraption as we came to a sliding door marked "Authorized Personnel Only." It opened, and she was wheeled into an antiseptic-looking hallway with another set of sliding doors beyond. "Good luck, we love you," we shouted as the doors slid shut.

We spent twelve hours, all told, in and around Waiting Room 3G at Emory University Hospital that day, November 1, 1995. Periodically we'd get an update from the Neurology Department's patient coordinator, Jim Stanton, who relayed information from the operating room that all was going fine. To ease our tension, Stanton assured us that Milly was patient 96 in Emory's pallidotomy program and that there had been no serious complications connected with the previous ninety-five. He also recounted pallidotomy lore: a Baptist minister, while undergoing the surgery, had "begun using the kind of language you're not supposed to hear from a Baptist minister." Another patient, a local Georgia resident, emerged from the surgery able to do a perfect, no-tremor Atlanta Braves tomahawk chop for the first time in years. I conveyed all of Stanton's upbeat reports on Milly's progress to friends and relatives by recording new messages on our home telephone answering machine.

I didn't necessarily believe what Stanton was saying about

Milly, however. I told Alex—a graduate student at NYU's film school, she was videotaping for a possible documentary—that if there were a "serious complication" in surgery, the doctors probably would not tell family members while it was under way for fear of causing panic in the waiting room. "I'm not pessimistic," I said. "It's just that I'll believe everything is okay when DeLong comes up here and tells us everything's okay." I remembered that I'd neglected to tell the doctors that Milly bruises easily. I worried that she might be prone to hemorrhaging. I also worried because she had not been able to sleep for two nights despite taking sleeping pills. Perhaps, I thought, lack of sleep would reduce her ability to cooperate during the surgery.

Fortunately, friends came to interrupt the worrying. Fred Barnes, my friend and colleague on *The McLaughlin Group*, joined us in the waiting room for a few hours on his way to Washington from visiting his parents in Florida. Jerry Leachman, an evangelist and leader of a men's religious fellowship that Fred had invited me to join a few years earlier, flew down from Washington for a few hours, too. We prayed together in the hospital chapel for Milly's safety and health. Alex fenced with Jerry about religion. "Christianity is not cool," she said. "You have an image problem with my generation—and I'm a moderate on this stuff." I told her that for someone to travel in a middle seat on Valuejet down to Atlanta to be with us was Christianity in action and that she should reconsider her values. I felt renewed chagrin that I had failed to provide my daughters with a religious education.

During the wait Alex and I had a conversation that was nearly as life-changing for me as anything else that has occurred during Milly's illness. Interviewing me for her film in a conference room, Alex asked me what would happen if Milly died in surgery. I said that I'd be bereft, but that I didn't know whether I'd fall apart, resume drinking, have a heart attack and die—or find some way to endure. I asked her what would happen to her. We turned the camera around, and she said that she and Andréa had had a long discussion about this the night before—their first ever, they realized.

"Andréa said that our family would fall apart and she would never see me or you again," Alex said. "She said that she'd never come home for Thanksgiving because you probably wouldn't bring her home."

I was shaken by this. "That's ridiculous," I said. "I'd want to feel closer to you kids than ever, though I don't know that you'd want to be close to me."

"Why?" Alex asked.

"Because Mom is the glue that holds our family together," I said.

Alex responded, "That's what Andréa said. And I said the same thing. 'Mom is the glue.' And if she was gone, everything would fall apart. I think I would maybe have to get married." She laughed nervously.

I said I thought I had drawn closer to the girls since I'd stopped drinking and since Milly had been sick, though I granted that most of the talk I had with them was "career talk," not "girl talk" like Milly could have. But I said, "Our family is not going to break up under any circumstances. I won't let it happen. If the worst happened in this operation, I would try to be as much of Mom as I possibly could be. But the worst is not going to happen. So let's not talk about this anymore."

Indeed, the worst did not happen, but I resolved on the spot to be as good a father in the future as I was trying to be a husband to Milly. I have been as good a father as I know how to be—calling the girls almost every day whether Milly instructs me to or not, seeing to it that they *are* home for holidays, hugging them often, praying for them every day, helping with money, and talking about their hopes and fears and souls as much—well, almost as much—as about their careers. The girls have had very different reactions to Milly's affliction. Alex will sit on a bed beside Milly and me and sob openly about how bad she feels. Andréa pulls away, talks clinically and practically about Milly's disease and confides her emotions only to her therapist. I notice her crying occasionally when she sees new evidence of Milly's decline, but she brushes away her tears if she knows someone is watching her.

I had asked Dr. DeLong whether I could be in the operating room for Milly's surgery. He told me firmly, "No." But I do have an idea of what happened in the operating room. I later witnessed an operation like Milly's, and I've seen videotapes of others. Milly was wheeled into Operating Room 15, a place surprisingly cluttered with books, papers, boxes, and spare surgical equipment as well as monitors and the operating table. The table was not flat; Milly's head was raised to a half-sitting position, and her legs were also elevated.

A four-foot frame was clamped to the table at head level and blue surgical sheets were attached to create a sterile environment from her forehead back. Her face, with the front of the halo bent outward over her nose and mouth, protruded from the front side of the sterile screen. The room was effectively divided in half. The front side was DeLong's side, dominated by electronic screens.

On the other side of the screen, the surgeon's side, a six-inch by three-inch swath of Milly's hair was shaved away as part of the preparation for surgery. A neurosurgery resident swabbed the area liberally with red disinfectant, then covered it over with layers of plastic prior to the arrival of the surgeon, Roy Bakay. Overweight, bearded, gruff, and prematurely gray—but commanding—Bakay was forty-six when he operated on Milly the first time. He'd been at Emory since 1982 after training in neurosurgery at the University of Washington and doing research at NIH. He met DeLong and his neurology associate, Jerrold Vitek, when they came to Emory from Hopkins in 1990. They'd done their first pallidotomy in 1992. Vitek and DeLong were both present for Milly's pallidotomy. Only Vitek was there for the operation I witnessed.

On Bakay's side, the patient's swathed head protruded through the sterile screen. Above her head, a complicated superstructure of frames was attached to the halo. Most prominent was a metal arc marked in centimeters and millimeters that could be moved forward and back and locked into the exact right place above her head. Attached to that was a black fitting for the microdrive, the $65,000 engine that would drive thinner-than-hair needles into her brain one millimeter at a time. The halo was bolted to the back of the operating table. The saying in brain surgery is that "a millimeter is a mile." There is no room for "play" or mistaken motion in any machine. Bakay attached the microdrive to its housing, then moved the arc out of the way temporarily as the surgery began. Bakay is celebrated, even notorious, at Emory for ensuring that everything is working correctly.

In the operation I witnessed, when Bakay cut the plastic coverings over the patient's head with scissors, exposing the scalp, he said, "This is the worst prep I've ever seen." He grabbed a razor blade and widened the area of exposure. He applied more disinfectant. Then he told the patient, "This will sting a little. It's a pain killer," and jabbed a surprisingly large needle into her scalp about three inches above the hairline. He touched the scalp to see whether numbing had begun, then jabbed again and again, deadening the entire area.

With a scalpel, he cut at a pre-marked place on her scalp and began using scissors to aggressively cut and pull the tissue away from the skull. An assistant clamped it back quickly. There was surprisingly little blood for such a large wound, about three inches in diameter.

Bakay abruptly left the sterile area, went around to the neurologist's side of the room, and studied the patient's MRI pictures, posted on a light-screen. He stripped off his outer surgical gown and gloves and dumped them into hampers.

When he returned to the sterile area, a nurse was waiting with fresh gloves—he wore three pairs much of the time—and a new surgical gown. He barked, "I don't know who set this up. The incision is about a mile behind where it's supposed to be." He went back to the patient and cut some more, now exposing about a four-inch-wide area on her skull. When I saw this operation I was thankful I'd been denied permission to watch Milly's. I would have been terrified, outraged at seeing errors, afraid to complain and afraid not to. The tension might have affected the outcome. For the surgery I watched, I was detached—and impressed with Bakay's refusal to accept less than perfect work. Out of earshot, a nurse called him "Mr. Grumpy." For the patient's sake, I was glad he had that attitude.

Once Bakay had made the incision he wanted, he moved the metal arc and the microdrive into place above the patient's scalp and fit a long, thin shaft with a protruding needle into the microdrive housing. He moved the needle above the exact spot where he wanted to open the skull and marked the spot with a pen, then moved the needle away again.

He swabbed on more disinfectant. Then he took a blue hand drill and began grinding at the skull. He stopped, chipped at the bone with a small chisel, and resumed drilling. At last he opened a hole twelve millimeters in diameter, about the size of a dime. Somehow it looked bigger to me, almost as big as a half-dollar. (In Milly's case, the hole and the operation were on the left side of her brain, so that the right side of her body would be affected.) When he had penetrated the skull, Bakay said, "We're now at the dura"—the tough, thin tissue that covers the brain. He used another small drill to penetrate it, then he moved the microdrive and needle into place above the hole, where fluid seemed to pulsate at the rate of heartbeats. "Are you ready down there?" he asked across the sterile screen. "Yeah," said Vitek.

The action moved to the neurologist's side. Vitek—or, in Milly's case, Vitek and DeLong taking turns—used a small handwheel to operate the microdrive, lowering the needle through the frontal lobe of the brain, where intelligence is centered, through the midbrain, and finally into the basal ganglia, which controls motion. The patient can feel none of this because the brain itself contains no nerve endings. The basal ganglia is located about three and a half inches deep in the brain. It contains the structures—striatum, globus pallidus, subthalamic nucleus, and substantia nigra—whose misfiring causes Parkinson's symptoms. The pallidotomy, by wounding the globus pallidus, is designed to restore fluidity of motion. In some cases a pallidotomy—or an operation on the subthalamic nucleii, as in Milly's later surgery—has also helped to restore a patient's balance.

Before the globus pallidus can be "burned," however, it must be precisely located and mapped. As Bakay and Vitek explained, an MRI does not provide a perfect, distortion-free picture of brain structures, so probes must be used to get a more accurate picture. It struck me that the pallidotomy "mapping and zapping" process resembles sonar-based submarine warfare as depicted in Tom

Clancy's *The Hunt for Red October*. In each case the doctor (captain) has a rough map of the terrain but must rely on sound readings to be sure of where he is and where his target is.

In the medical case, the tip of the needle penetrating the patient's brain contains a tiny electrode that picks up the distinct electrical signals transmitted by various kinds of cells. The signals are converted into sounds and electronic graph readings in the operating room. The sounds crackle like radio static. Just as a good sonar operator can distinguish one class of enemy submarine from another, Vitek and DeLong can distinguish one part of the brain from another. Vitek compares the process to riding in a train through Europe wearing a blindfold: "You can tell where you are by the languages you hear." The neurologist's side of the operating room is dark during the mapping, and Vitek, wearing earphones, reads out reports to technicians who use flashlights to record his findings on a graph sheet.

The globus pallidus is the size of a small plum, with an internal and external structure, the GPI and the GPE. It's the GPI that must be damaged at precise points. These are located by having the patient move limbs, fingers, eyes, eyelids, and tongue, each setting off a distinctive electronic signal. Vitek and DeLong can move the electrode up and down into the brain structures one micron (one-tenth of a millimeter) at a time, a distance no deeper than a cell. But to move to different planes or lines of attack, they have to extract the needle and reinsert it. In a pallidotomy, special care has to be taken to avoid damaging the optic nerve or the brain's internal capsule, which can render the patient blind or paralyzed.

In the operation I saw, as Vitek mapped, Bakay periodically came around to study the MRI picture and calculate new courses for penetration. Then he would regown and reglove, return to his post, adjust the magnifying lenses attached to his eyeglasses, and change the position of the microdrive for the next insertion.

In Milly's case, the three doctors made nine separate penetrations of the brain on different parallel planes. The average is four to five, according to DeLong. On the first mapping pass they found the GPI but wanted to explore further. On the second and third, moving the needle's angle, they hit the GPE and the striatum, not the GPI. On the fourth they hit no significant cells at all. On the fifth they found the optic track—doing it no damage, fortunately—but not the globus pallidus. On the sixth they got good readings from the internal globus pallidus. Having found the target again, they went in three more times with another sort of electrode—this time not to listen and map but to inflict lesions with a tiny heat probe.

When the damage was done, with hoped-for beneficial results, the main action in the operating room reverted to Bakay, who installed a hard plastic plug in the hole in the patient's skull and then, with a resident assisting, unclamped and meticulously stitched up the patient's wound. Then he installed dozens of staples into the scalp and covered the whole with a large white bandage. From start to finish, Milly's first ordeal lasted from 8:00 A.M., when the halo pins were drilled into her head, until 6:00 P.M., when she left for the recovery room. The surgery itself had lasted seven hours.

DeLong came to see us in the waiting room and said he thought he had noticed improvement in her fluidity of motion. And he told us that she had been "a star" in the operating room. "She kept worrying that she wouldn't do things right," he said, "but I told her she won the prize." There was no problem with hemorrhaging or any other complication. The doctors had put her to sleep while closing her wound and removing her head-gear, he said. We could see her in an hour or two. Milly's NIH doctor, Leo Verhagen, had been in the operating room, and he, too, came in to report to us that everything had gone well. DeLong said that he could not predict how long any good effects from the surgery would last. At this point we were all ecstatic merely that Milly had come through the surgery and that there had been "improvement." We were not surprised that she had behaved like a heroine.

Milly's first words were, "Alex, turn off that camera. I look terrible." We all laughed at her vanity and told her that, to us, she looked beautiful. And in spite of bandages and dark circles under her eyes, she did. Her forehead seemed less wrinkled, and her face looked more relaxed. I had her grab my fingers with her right hand. Her grip seemed significantly stronger than it had been before the operation. As we left the room to let Milly rest for the night, Alex asked, "Well, what do you think?" I said, "I think, terrific."

Milly and I were deeply invested in the success of this operation. The week before going to Atlanta, Milly had said she hoped that she wouldn't freeze anymore, that she would be able to walk, that her posture would improve and she wouldn't fall. "I want to be perfect," she'd said, "but the doctors say I won't be. But I'll take 80 or 90 percent." I said, "I'd be deeply grateful to have 80 percent of the Old Milly back." I hoped, on the basis of something De-Long had told me, that some of Milly's indomitable personality and fast wit might return because, with her body functioning better, she'd be less depressed. "Depression saps mental energy," he had contended. We were all talking guardedly, but somewhere inside we harbored a vision of Milly whole again—able to walk and drive, work and argue, boss and laugh and give good advice.

The first indications were good. The next morning DeLong and Vitek got Milly out of bed, and she and I danced briefly around the room. Her balance wasn't perfect, but it seemed improved, and I thought she moved less haltingly than before the surgery. She was back on Sinemet, and she performed better on all the tests in the classic neurological exam. Later Alex and Andréa arrived with the rest of Milly's army of visitors, now joined by Jill Schuker. Milly's first solid food was brought in, and she ate and drank without any sign of tremor or stiffness. We all agreed that her appetite was much better. Jill said, making a toasting motion, "A success. A new beginning. A new sense of normal." Milly responded, "I don't know. I'm still afraid." I took the group out shopping, buying each person a gift to commemorate the occasion. For Milly, we bought a half-dozen smart hats and caps that could cover her bandages for the trip back home and for as long as it took for her hair to grow back. I tried to get Milly to keep her hair short and let it go all white, like her sister Alex's. But when we got back to Washington, she immediately bought an expensive dark brown wig. And when her hair grew in she dyed the white away—determined, she said, not to look older than I did. Even though we hoped she would be liberated from many Parkinson's symptoms, Milly anticipated that tremor might make it hard for her to put on makeup, so she painfully had eyeliner tattooed above and below her lashes.

The pallidotomy produced some immediate improvement, and we judged it a net success. But it did not bring back the Old Milly. To the good, her lips stopped involuntarily pursing, which had made her feel sick. She no longer froze in a chair. She could "scoot" and turn in bed. Her grip remained strong. But Milly's voice kept losing power. She did not become less depressed. And she did not stop falling.

The old pattern resumed: some days, she could walk around the house safely by herself or using a walker. In 1996, when a PBS crew filmed her being examined at NIH for a documentary I did on the politics of medical research, she walked around the hallways on my arm with only a brief stumble. But other times, at home and away, she collapsed forward or to the side and was unable to break her fall. The emergency room visits recurred, and the stitches. One day when Andréa was home from medical school, Milly had almost reached the bottom of the stairs when she suddenly fell forward, hitting her head on a wall. She was stunned and couldn't remember our dog's name. We put our three-story house on the market and signed a contract on a one-story rambler. But Milly, typically, refused to set a realistic price on the house that she loved, and in a down-market, we got no offers for more than a year. I lived in renewed fear that she would fall down the stairs again and injure herself severely.

My anxiety—both immediate and long-term—deepened when I visited Mo Udall's hospital room in 1996. *The Washingtonian* magazine asked me to write an article on Parkinson's after Attorney General Janet Reno announced she had been diagnosed the previous year. She refused to be interviewed, though. I was also turned down by the Reverend Billy Graham, then misdiagnosed as having Parkinson's. (It later turned out he had hydrocephalus, which could be relieved by a fluid-draining shunt.) So I made Mo Udall—and Milly—the central characters of my article. I got help from Udall's wife, Norma.

Long considered the funniest man in Congress and one of the strongest liberals and environmentalists, Udall was diagnosed in 1976, at the age of fifty-three, while he was running for president. He kept it secret at the time and was helped in doing so by NIH's Dr. Tom Chase, later Milly's doctor. Chase has helped other celebrities hide their Parkinson's as well. L-dopa kept Udall largely symptom-free until the early 1980s, when his six-foot-five frame began to stoop, his head began to shake, and his facial muscles began to freeze into "the mask," a common Parkinson's symptom that Milly does not share. Udall's speech, like Milly's did later, became progressively slurred. His personality also changed, though not the way hers did. He became forgetful, retelling jokes everyone had heard before, even the same evening. By the late 1980s he was experiencing mild hallucinations, as some Parkinson's patients do in response to L-dopa. Norma said he thought he saw a little white dog ducking around their house, though they didn't have one.

As time went on, Udall could barely get into and out of a car. He had difficulty getting words out. Either the medicine or the disease turned his internal clock around, so that he'd stay up all night pacing the house and be dead tired the next day, when he was supposed to be alert in chairing the House Interior Committee. He couldn't cut his food and eventually had to be fed. He did not suffer from depression, according to his wife. "He'd kid," she said. "When he couldn't get out of the car, he'd say, 'Look at me, the star athlete.' It was black humor."

Udall announced after his reelection in 1990 that he wouldn't run again, but he did not make it to the end of his term. In January 1991, tired of watching an NFL playoff game, he decided to go upstairs to bed. "See ya later," he told Norma. The Udalls' townhouse had an elevator, but he hated to use it because if he leaned against the door, it would stop between floors and he couldn't make it start. Besides, of all the afflictions of Parkinson's, the one he didn't seem to have was trouble climbing stairs.

Norma said she heard him mount four or five stairs. Then she heard him yell—and crash. She ran to find his head covered with blood. He had suffered a concussion and broken four ribs, a collarbone, and a shoulder blade. He spent weeks in intensive care, then went to the Veterans Administration hospital about three miles north of the Capitol. He was unable to swallow and was fed through a tube into his stomach. He never returned to Congress and formally resigned in May 1991 after thirty years of service. "See ya later" were the last clear words anyone ever heard Udall utter.

When I walked into Udall's hospital room with Norma, he was asleep. He looked younger than his seventy-three years. The room was plastered with photos from his pro basketball days, presidential campaign posters, and other political mementos. A guest book indicated he'd been visited by First Ladies Barbara Bush and Hillary Rodham Clinton and by many House and Senate colleagues—most frequently by Senator John McCain, whom Udall had befriended, even though he was a Republican, when McCain was a freshman Arizona congressman and the most junior member of the Interior Committee.

When Norma woke him up, telling him that he had a visitor, Udall looked at me with what seemed to be recognition and a small smile, the way an experienced pol does with a constituent whose name he doesn't remember. I started regaling him with the latest political news: President Clinton's election-year State of the Union address, Newt Gingrich's diving poll ratings. For five minutes or so he seemed to brighten and his eyes suggested comprehension. Then he fell back to sleep.

I could not tell whether he understood anything. Norma said that she couldn't tell either whether he comprehended what she said and read to him. *If he does,* I thought, *it's a terrifying situation: he is trapped in his body, unable to connect with other people.* I hoped that his mind had closed down, but I knew that Milly's had not. While there were differences in their cases, they were frighteningly similar. Udall, when he fell, had had Parkinson's for fifteen years. At the time I visited him Milly had had it for nine. At a minimum, I had to see to it that she did not fall down stairs again. So I insisted that we get what we could for our house—$100,000 less than we had hoped for, as it turned out—and move to a condominium apartment in an embassy neighborhood, Kalorama, near downtown D.C. I love the area, which has the elegant atmosphere of Upper East Side Manhattan, and the apartment has high ceilings, a fireplace, and a balcony. But Milly hates it because she misses our old home and because the new one is a symbol of her incapacity.

Moving may have prevented a catastrophic fall, but it did not prevent falls. We merely switched emergency rooms, from Suburban Hospital in Maryland to Georgetown and Sibley in D.C. Milly kept trying to get around with walkers and often succeeded one day, only to tumble the next. In early 1997, she fell in the bathroom, splitting her lip and breaking her nose. She needed plastic surgery to repair the damage, and she decided that, since her nose was going to be operated on, she would get the reduction she had always wanted. I couldn't possibly refuse. After that operation she looked truly ghastly. She had two black eyes and bloody bandages pushed up her nostrils. But this operation was a success.

We'd bought a wheelchair even before we moved, but Milly resisted using it. Then one Saturday morning an event occurred that fulfilled one of Milly's terrible early fears about Parkinson's. I left the house to run a quick errand, telling Milly sternly to stay in bed until I got back. If she had to go to the toilet, I said, she was to use a portable commode that we had next to the bed, not try to get to the bathroom. Shortly after I left Jill called. When Milly reached for the phone, she rolled off the bed, and her head became wedged between the mattress and a handrail we'd attached to the bed to help her rise. Milly fumbled with the phone and screamed to Jill that she couldn't move. She was in the same situation as the Neurology Center patient whose plight had so moved her years before. Jill rushed to our apartment, only to find the door locked. Just as she was getting ready to call the police to have it knocked down, if necessary, I returned. Milly was shaken and sobbing as I got her back into bed. It was clear that she could not be left alone, ever, and we began looking for personal assistants. About the same time it became obvious that Milly would fall if she even tried to use a walker, so she settled for being pushed around in a wheelchair.

Other symptoms also worsened. Her voice kept losing resonance and volume, though she still could be understood. The tightness in her lips and face returned. She often had swollen feet. Her handwriting became almost completely illegible. She became incontinent. At first this problem seemed to occur only when she coughed, and a urologist said it was not unusual for postmenopausal women. Milly had an operation designed to correct the problem—and at the same time got a thinning tummy tuck— and then took medicine. But the problem worsened, causing embarrassment and a search for appropriate pads and protective underwear. Because she had no sense of balance, she could not change herself, so I did it in the months before we got full-time help. All this was a humiliation to a woman who'd always been so meticulous about her personal appearance and so determined in her independence. It is also a continuing inconvenience, trying to decide at a crowded airport or a theater whether to wheel Milly into a men's bathroom or a women's. I complain about this. She gets upset. On one such occasion, as we tried to negotiate a too-small stall in a women's bathroom at Midway Airport in Chicago, she whispered to me, "I hate my life."

The pallidotomy did nothing to ease Milly's depression. Neither did Prozac or Zoloft, which marginally worsened it because they were not only ineffective but caused Milly to gain weight. When I interviewed her for the PBS show she said, "I can't do anything for myself because I can't stand. So I have to have somebody here all the time. They have to clean house because I can't do it. I'll fall. I can't wash dishes. I can't dress myself. I can't pick up my pants myself. Someone has to go into the bathroom with me. I've lost my dignity. People have to help me do everything. Even eat—I can't cut my meat."

She sobbed. "It makes me feel terrible because I have to depend on you for everything," she told me. "I'm completely lost. I haven't got any independence. I used to drive my own car. Now you have to help me in and out of the car. You have to go with me every place, and if you sit me down I have to stay seated there because I'll fall if I get up.

"Every day something new happens to me, something else I can't do. Something else. Something else. Make another adjustment. The worst is that I have to ask permission for things. I'm going to be a baby. A baby—that's what I am. I can't do anything. I have to ask permission to go to the refrigerator, permission to get a book, permission to go to the bathroom."

About the pallidotomy she said, with a little laugh, "Well, they put an umbrella or a lampshade on your head. And then they drill a hole in your head, and they go into your brain and hit something. You're awake the whole time and doing different things for them." She got serious. "The operation didn't work. Some things are worse because of it. My handwriting got worse. My balance didn't improve. And I'm constipated all the time."

I asked her whether there was anything on the medical horizon that gave her hope. "I don't see anything. I see a dead future. They aren't going to find anything. Maybe someday, but not for me. I have no hope."

I asked her whether she was depressed. "This depression really owns me," she said. "I want to die before I become a vegetable. I think I have about three years because it seems to be going rapidly, the deterioration. I think I'm going to be Mo Udall in three years." She started to cry again. "I'm probably going to die. I want to live. I don't want to be like Mo Udall. I don't want to be kept alive."

She wanted to live, but not like this. So in 1998 we began looking again for medical options. Joan Samuelson consulted all the leading neurologists she knew and made a list of who was doing what kind of procedure. I started calling them to ask what we might do. At the University of Colorado, Dr. Curt Freed said that fetal transplantation still wasn't ready. In any event, he said, Milly would not fit into his study protocol because she had already had a pallidotomy. Dr. Ole Isaacson at Harvard raised the same issue about a study he was involved in, using fetal cells from pigs. Two other promising theoretical areas, neural growth factors and genetic engineering, were nowhere near ready for trial on humans.

The newest practical thing being done was deep-brain stimulation (DBS) of one of the structures of the basal ganglia—the globus pallidus or the subthalamic nucleus (STN). This involved implantation of a pacemaker-like device in the brain—and a battery under the flesh of the chest—to modulate the hyperactive circuits. The operation had been performed most often in Europe

but was also being done in Canada, at the University of Kansas—
and by DeLong and Vitek at Emory. Milly and I went to Kansas
City for an exam, and doctors there said they thought she might
benefit from the surgery. We briefly considered going to Liège in
Belgium after a Washington friend said she could arrange for us to
stay with the royal family there. Instead, because of DeLong, we
went back to Emory.

We saw him in September, and Milly begged him to schedule
the surgery—and to install an electrode not just on one side of
her brain but on both sides at the same time. She wanted a decisive outcome. DeLong said that he thought she might benefit
from stimulation of the STN, but he said that the Emory team
had never done a bilateral procedure before and that he'd have to
check with Bakay and Vitek to see whether it made sense. After
we went back home, Milly told me over and over that only a double stimulation would do. I relayed her wishes to DeLong, and he
finally said that he'd do it—on October 26, a Monday.

Milly and I arrived in Atlanta on the Thursday before, and she
underwent preliminary checks on Friday. All weekend I drove back
and forth to the airport to collect a small army of family and well-
wishers who assembled to be with her, including Alex and Andréa,
Lori, Joan Samuelson, Dr. Verhagen, and Milly's foster mother Annie. Of course, we took everyone shopping, too. Lori, who is as
close to Milly as a real sister, told me later that while I was off doing something, Milly confided in Annie how frightened and desperate she was. The first operation had done little lasting good.
She hoped for a miracle with this one, but feared it would not happen. She was furious at the endless doctor visits, tests, medicines,
and trips to the hospital that she had to endure. "Why me?" she
cried, and tried to figure out what terrible wrong she had committed to be condemned to this.

"Here she was," Lori told me, "blaming herself, when she had been nothing except a tower of strength to everyone in crisis all her life. Milly's love is boundless. It has no end. I think it feeds her own need to be loved and cherished by others, but it comes out as pure generosity." Annie tried to comfort Milly by telling her stories of crises in her own life that her daughter, Lori, had never heard before. "True to form, Milly was so touched by someone else's pain that she put aside her own," Lori told me.

On the day of the operation we gathered in the same room where we had waited out the first operation, 3G. But this time DeLong said I could accompany Milly for the installation of the halo and the MRI to follow, though not for the operation.

The prep room looked familiar, like a hospital emergency room with screened-off areas in which many patients were being readied for surgery of various kinds. Milly complained not at all as an attendant cut off most of the hair on the front half of her head and shaved a wide swath. The aide also cut and shaved spots at the rear of her head. Then a nurse, warning Milly that it would hurt, stuck needles in her forehead and in the back of her head. When the skin was numb, she fitted the halo over Milly's head and began turning the four sharp screws on its mount toward Milly's head and then into her skin. She turned each with a small wrench tight into Milly's scalp. It was painful for me to watch, but Milly took it like a heroine. She was a veteran, after all.

Then, with the halo around her head, she was wheeled to an elevator and downstairs for an MRI. Milly has been inside this massive machine dozens of times over the years, and she still detests MRIs because they are so confining and noisy. She usually wants me with her, and I was glad that I could be there this time, holding her leg, massaging her feet, and telling her amid the clanking how much I loved her.

Afterward she disappeared again into the operating room—this time for more than twelve hours. Stanton reappeared to give us periodic updates on Milly's progress—again, all positive. This time I was more inclined to believe him, although I did not share Milly's hopes that the implants would be the miracle that she yearned for. My wildest dreams would be fulfilled, I thought, if there were just some improvement in her balance, if she could perhaps use a walker again. Jerry Leachman once more flew down to Atlanta to be with us and to pray for Milly's well-being. As during the pallidotomy, I left messages on our home answering machine reporting that Milly was doing fine.

Again, I know something about what was happening in the operating room. The surgery I witnessed later was a DBS implant in a woman's subthalamic nucleus. Much of the operation was similar to a pallidotomy except that the target was different and the purpose was not to damage the organ. After three mapping tracks, Bakay installed a millimeter-thick tube into the microdrive. Inside was a thinner wire with four electrical contact points on the end, all crowded into a space of three millimeters.

About the time the actual implant was to occur, everyone in the operating room had to don lead vests as technicians wheeled a huge fluoroscope into the room to give Bakay and Vitek a real-time picture of the insertion. The machine was positioned on Bakay's side of the sterile barrier and aimed at the woman's head from two sides. A monitor showed the long tube extending into the patient's brain. Bakay told me that the purpose of having this picture was to make sure that when the guide tube was removed the electrical lead did not move with it and leave the target point.

I asked Vitek whether it wouldn't make sense to have a machine—an MRI or a super-fluoroscope—that could guide the surgeon and the neurologists during the entire operation. He said that some hospitals did have such a device—including the University of Minnesota, where he'd received his M.D. and Ph.D.—but not yet Emory. I said that, as things were, "what you do here definitely is rocket science, but it is also art." He agreed with that. And to prove the point, the fluoroscope picture showed an unwanted bend at the end of the electrode wire in the patient's brain. Bakay delicately manipulated the microdrive to straighten it and put the lead exactly where it was supposed to be in the STN, a structure that's even smaller than the globus pallidus, about the size of a large pea or small grape. When it was in place, Vitek sent impulses of various voltages down the wire and tested the patient for responses. He asked her to move her fingers, hands, feet, and legs at each voltage—one to five—and tried out various combinations of contacts. The patient reported feeling dizzy at three volts, but that subsided.

When Vitek believed he had the optimal setting, Bakay and a resident closed the wound, as in the pallidotomy. But in this case a wire extended through the plug in the top of the head. The patient, awake throughout the STN implant, was given a general anesthesia. Then Bakay made a two-inch opening in her chest just below the collarbone. He installed a two-inch-square battery and, using another guide tube, ran the wire under the scalp, behind the patient's ear and down into the chest, connecting it to the battery. Then he sewed her up for removal to the recovery room.

The surgery I watched lasted from 9:45 A.M., when Bakay made his first incision, to 4:30 P.M., when the patient received her last stitches. This was just a one-side STN implant, however. Milly received two implants. And before they installed them, De-Long, Vitek, and Bakay did twelve mapping tracks, seven on her left side and five on the right. Milly's surgery lasted until 10:00 P.M., more than twelve hours. It was an ordeal for her and also for

Bakay. DeLong and Vitek, when they came to the waiting room to report, made it clear that Bakay had not appreciated the task. When he arrived I thanked him profusely.

The doctors warned that Milly's brain had undergone a lot of penetration. So, they said, if the operation achieved results, they might be longer taking hold than for the pallidotomy. This warning didn't prepare us, however, for the scare that followed: Milly did not wake up on schedule from the anesthesia. "This happens," DeLong said, trying to be reassuring. "The brain takes time to recover." DeLong did not use the word *coma*, but that is what we feared he meant. All of us in the waiting room found ourselves begging God to let Milly be okay.

Sometime after midnight, we were allowed to see her briefly in the intensive care unit. Andréa lovingly caressed her mother's forehead and softly called on her over and over to wake up. Andréa asked her to move a finger. She put her finger in Milly's hand and encouraged her to squeeze it. Milly did not respond. We were ushered out and went back to the waiting room. We stayed there nearly until dawn, hoping for some positive word, but we were merely told that Milly was "sleeping." We went back to our hotel for a few hours, reassuring each other that Milly would be awake when we returned. None of us slept that night, however.

Milly was better the next morning. She was alert. She could be understood, though her voice was soft. But she was having difficulty swallowing and had to continue receiving nutrients intravenously. She got out of bed and tried to walk, but there did not seem to be any improvement in her balance. This operation seemed less successful than the pallidotomy. On Wednesday she was able to eat soft foods, which was a huge relief. But DeLong surprised and disturbed me by saying that she would have to stay in the hospital for several days of recovery and after that would need to be transferred to a rehabilitation hospital for physical and occupational therapy. Her brain had undergone more probing and stress than during the pallidotomy, he said, and she needed extra time and help recovering.

I started scrambling—first to find the appropriate hospital and get insurance clearances, and then to figure out whether I could still do all the work I was committed to. The 1998 congressional elections were less than a week away, and I had lined up a horrendous schedule that I'd thought I could handle based on Milly's quick rebound after the pallidotomy. It was easy enough to phone in from the hospital the two columns I had to write Tuesday and Thursday for *Roll Call*—one on the Monica Lewinsky scandal and one on the forthcoming elections. But then I was supposed to be in New York Friday to tape the Fox News show *The Beltway Boys*, which I had started with Fred Barnes that summer, departing from *The McLaughlin Group* after sixteen years. And I was supposed to stay in New York for an election rehearsal Saturday morning and Fox News Sunday. I was also scheduled to make a speech in New Orleans Sunday night.

Andréa and Alex said they'd stay in Atlanta with Milly while I traveled, and Jill arrived to be with them. I canceled the New Orleans speech but flew to New York on Friday, then flew back to Atlanta Sunday afternoon. I spent Sunday and Monday with Milly and flew back to New York Tuesday morning, did election commentary Tuesday night, and flew back to Atlanta Wednesday morning on next to no sleep. I wrote my column on the plane and phoned it to *Roll Call* from the hospital. I checked Milly out of the hospital that afternoon. As we drove to the airport she was sporting one of a new set of hats we'd bought. Back in Washington we drove to the National Rehabilitation Hospital and checked her in.

It remained all too obvious that the surgery had done Milly

little good at all and might have done harm. Again, to the good, the dyskinesia in Milly's face eased, relaxing the muscles in her lips and forehead. But there was no improvement in her balance. Her voice volume and ability to articulate were worse. She could no longer chew food and continued to have difficulty swallowing. While Milly was at NRH for two weeks, I bought various microphones, amplifiers, and portable speakers, which I hoped would allow her voice to be heard. But she still could not be understood because she could not articulate words well. She could not swallow her medicine with water. She'd gulp and the liquid would go down her windpipe. She risked aspirating the pills, so she had to begin taking her medicine with applesauce. The rehab hospital taught her how to move from a bed to her wheelchair and from the wheelchair to a toilet.

We went through one last procedure that we fervently hoped would improve Milly's basic condition. A specialist from Medtronic, the company that makes the DBS system, came to NIH to adjust the voltage and other settings of the electrodes. Watching, I prayed that some new combination would suddenly produce a transformation. He worked for three hours, repeatedly moving a magnetic wand above the control system embedded in Milly's chest. He tried one permutation after another—three volts on the right side, two on the left, top lead on the right and bottom on the left, and so on. But in the end he concluded that DeLong and Vitek had established the optimal settings in the first place. There was no longer much hope that Milly could avoid being rendered a permanent invalid by Parkinson's.

The prospect was made harder to bear by the astounding success at Emory experienced by a woman named Sybil Guthrie, who was the subject of a widely watched *Dateline NBC* segment in 1999. Before her first STN implant, Mrs. Guthrie had many of

Milly's symptoms. She was confined to a wheelchair and had difficulty eating and speaking. She suffered severe tremor and had to be helped getting dressed. Her face was freezing into a "mask." After one implant operation, she was able to walk and talk slowly and the tremor subsided on one side. She had a second STN implant some months later, and the transformation was profound. She laughed. She spoke clearly. And in the last scene of the segment she ran freely, beaming, through her backyard. When Milly and I watched the segment together, we were glad for Mrs. Guthrie, but the question of Milly's that I could not answer was: "Why didn't that happen to me?"

We watched this together. We do as much together as we possibly can. But just before Milly's first surgery she'd said, "If you get sick, you are alone. Nobody can be with you. Nobody knows how you feel. Nobody wants to be with you that long. You are alone. No matter how much people love you, you are alone." I love her profoundly, and I am determined not to let her suffer alone.

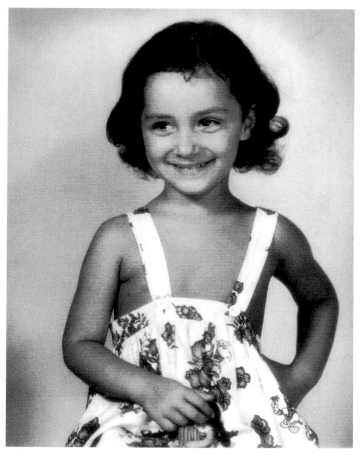

Millicent Martinez, age 3

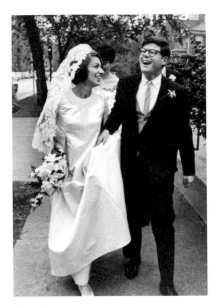

October 7, 1967,
Hyde Park, Chicago

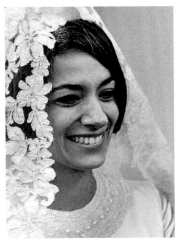

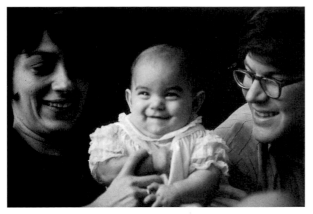

Milly and me with baby Alexandra

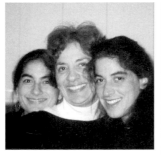

Milly with our daughters,
Alex and Andréa (1991)

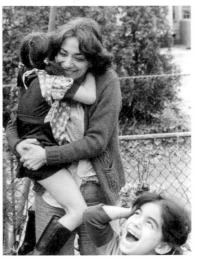

Milly with Andréa (in her arms)
and Alex

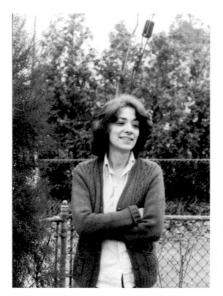

In the back yard at the first house we owned in Washington

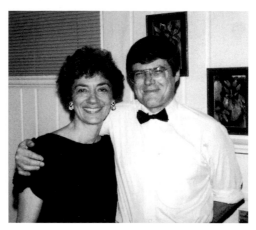

At Andréa's 16th birthday party, July 1986

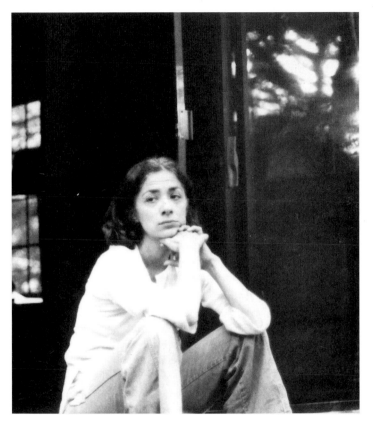

The Old Milly

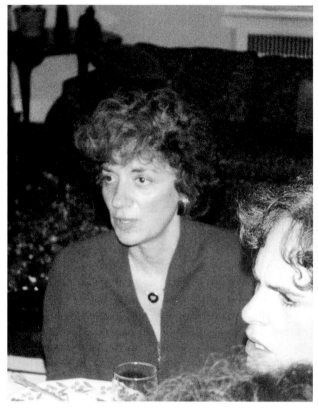

Milly at a Thanksgiving dinner at our home in Chevy
Chase, Md., with Judy Siegel post-diagnosis

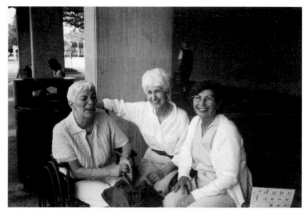

Milly (in wheelchair) with her sisters, Alex and Lori

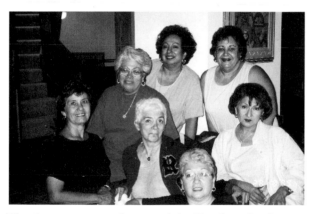

The August 2000 gathering of the "Roulettes" at Lori Long's house: Milly (seated center) surrounded by (from left) Nancy Chavez Gomez, Helen Metoyer, Adele Hernandez, Pat Gonzalez, Eva Velarde, and Mona Reyes

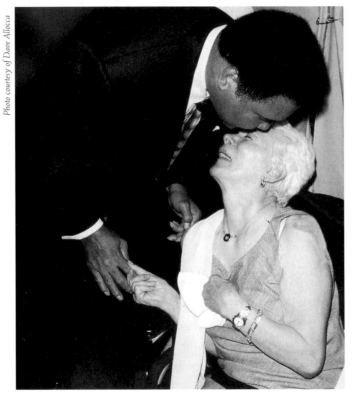

Milly meets Muhammad Ali at a reception for Ali and
Michael J. Fox during the Republican National Convention in Philadelphia, August 2000

5

The New Mort

Much as it was a family ritual to spend Christmas with the Wheelers in Vermont, each summer Milly and I rented a beach house for two weeks in Delaware, Virginia, or North Carolina. Finally we built a cottage in Bethany Beach, Delaware. Some years the Wheelers would vacation with us, some years it was the Longs, and one time my mother visited. On that occasion, in a rented rowboat on a saltwater pond, I got a glimpse of why I was the person I was.

To get from the rental shack to the pond, I had to row about a quarter of a mile along a narrow channel. My mother, Genevieve, then about sixty-five—now she's eighty-seven—was riding in the boat. The other people in our group were already at the pond trying to catch crabs. By the time we entered the pond I was tired but we still had about a hundred yards to cover to join the others. My mother said, "Here, I'll row, too." So she took one oar, and I took the other. We started rowing, but we didn't get anywhere. The boat kept going around in a circle, the bow turning in my direction. I rowed harder, but she rowed harder still. The boat kept going in a circle. Finally I said, "Hey, this is not a competition! It's supposed to be cooperation!"

Eventually we got to where we were going. My mother wasn't even aware of what she'd done. Competitiveness just came naturally to her. She'd been a swimmer at the University of Illinois in the days when men's teams traveled to other Big Ten schools for their meets, but women swam in their own pools and matched times with the other team by telegraph. To this day my mother is furious at that inequity. But the consequence was that I grew up in an atmosphere of rivalry and comparison—with my brother, with my peers, with my images of who I was and ought to be and what I could do and should.

My mother is not to blame for my neuroses. After a certain age I became responsible for them. But I grew up self-absorbed and dissatisfied with myself. I stayed that way into adulthood. I envied people with natural abilities—high IQs, artistic talent, winning personalities, good looks, athletic prowess—and felt that I was condemned to mediocre above-averageness. I dismissed the gifts that God and other people (including my parents) gave me—good health, "the gift of gab," a good education, an early start in the right profession—and fixated on what I didn't have.

From childhood on I spent countless hours vainly drawing up self-improvement lists. The "do" items always started with "lose weight," followed by "exercise daily," "learn languages," "read books," "quit smoking," and, later, "quit drinking." For a long time I carried in my billfold a list of the attributes by which I wanted to be defined—"strong, honest, deep, independent, humane." I didn't include "diligent" because that was a given. Had I ever actually improved myself into my ideal, the resulting person would have been a lofty loner, not someone who mixed it up easily with people. I somehow thought intimacy was beyond my power. Of course, I talked to other people and tried to act friendly toward them. I wanted to be liked—to be loved, in fact. But I was convinced that likability and lovability were characteristics I simply wasn't born with and had no idea how to cultivate. Much as paranoids create enemies, narcissists have a hard time being popular.

Terrified of failure, I achieved a fair amount of professional success—largely, I now understand, because I was blessed with generous mentors who gave me opportunities. But for years I had it fixed in my head that my talent and performance gave me a lifetime grade in the 89.9th percentile among my peers—a B+. I feared that at any moment I could lose what I had to someone who ranked in the 95th percentile in brains or other talent, an A+. I constantly, stupidly, ranked people by percentile, and I found it hard to bond with anyone significantly higher or lower than I, or with bosses. There were a few things I had done in my life that I considered unqualifiedly first-class. One was marrying Milly. Another was asking penetrating questions in a 1984 presidential debate with eighty million people watching on TV. But most of the time the message I heard as I obsessively judged myself was "Not Good Enough."

Milly's diagnosis changed me. When it became clear in 1988 that she had Parkinson's, I said to myself, "This is one thing in your life you are going to do right." I meant that I was determined to be a loving husband and to help Milly fight the disease. I certainly did not want to stop being professionally successful, but I decided that my career was now secondary as the purpose of my life. I did not know what helping Milly fight Parkinson's might involve, and I did not want to know. People recommended a newly published book, *Mainstay* by Maggie Strong, described as the bible for spouses of the chronically ill. But I refused to read it. I was afraid that if I had a forecast of how bad things could become I might shrink from the ordeal. I figured I would simply deal with whatever happened, as it happened.

This has become my philosophy of life: do the best you can playing the hand you are dealt, and ask God's help every single step of the way. I call this Christian stoicism. It could just as easily be Jewish or Buddhist, and my research into the great Stoics, Marcus Aurelius and Epictetus, suggests that my ideas do not align exactly with theirs. Epictetus says that in the great drama of life it is up to "the Author" to give you a role to play and that your job is to "act well the given part." That much tracks with what I believe. But Epictetus seems to demand absolute perfectionism in playing the part through total control of one's will. My mantra is more lenient: do the best you can. I repeat it to myself constantly—almost as often as I say, "Please, God." "Do your best" permits some falling short of an ideal performance, but it still creates an inner high standard. The penalty for violating it is shame.

My standard for myself with Milly has been to be consistently loving, caring, patient, and supportive. On several occasions, though, I have yelled at her—especially when she tried some risky walking maneuver, crashed, and hurt herself. Especially in the years before she was confined to a wheelchair—but occasionally since then—when I left the room to walk the dog or get something in the kitchen, I'd tell her to stay seated and not try anything adventuresome while I was out. Then I'd return and find her splayed on the floor, sometimes with a cut lip or bruised forehead. Even though she was in pain and deserved comfort, I'd explode in fear and anger: "Goddammit, I *told* you not to do that!" And I'd grab her, pull her roughly to her feet, and put her down hard in her chair or wheelchair. I have never caused her any injury or physical pain, but she has looked at me as though she feared that I might. Every time, within seconds, I've been overwhelmed with remorse and asked to be forgiven.

I call my stoicism Christian partly because I grew up a Protestant and feel comfortable in that tradition. I do not consider Christianity by any means the exclusive path to God, but it is the one I am familiar with. And it has become an increasingly important part of my life, beginning when I quit drinking and joined Alcoholics Anonymous, one of the main principles of which is to yield one's will to that of a Higher Power.

My former television tormentor, John McLaughlin, who once was a Jesuit priest, often jibed that I was "a pilgrim" on a never-ending political and theological quest. He was right. I was a liberal during the civil rights era but could not remain one when I thought that liberals were abandoning millions of innocents around the world to communism and apologizing for criminals who terrorized the poor. Yet I couldn't side with conservatives, who seemed to argue that it was just too bad if people couldn't make it on their own. After being attacked as wishy-washy for sometimes taking one side and sometimes another—and fearing there was no room for somebody like me in the talking-head trade—I finally found my political home in New Democrat moderation. Gratifyingly, enough viewers, readers, editors, and TV executives seem to appreciate non-ideological commentary that I stay employed.

My spiritual pilgrimage commenced out of a combination of professional failure, personal trauma, and the lessons of AA. When I became *Newsweek*'s Washington bureau chief in 1985 I had visions of being editor someday, even though management was not my calling. I spent eighteen months in almost constant agony and left feeling defeated and savagely depressed. The most natural thing would have been for me to continue anesthetizing myself with alcohol, but it was a blessing that Milly had just then succeeded in convincing me to quit drinking. I joined AA a month after leaving *Newsweek*. AA promised a kind of redemption and deliverance that I had always yearned for—the experience of Scrooge on Christmas morning in my favorite story, Dickens's "A Christmas Carol."

After a month of attending AA meetings almost daily and reading its literature, members of *The McLaughlin Group* traveled to Mexico in December 1986 with our spouses to deliver a panel presentation. I awoke on a Sunday morning with an unmistakable feeling of self-identity as a believing Christian. It was not a born-again experience. There was no vision, no presence. And yet I think of it as a conversion. I felt that I knew where I wanted to go spiritually, where home was for me.

The spiritual pilgrimage continues, however, partly because I cannot answer Milly's agonized, unanswerable questions—"Why did God do this to me?" and, "Why is God punishing me?" I joined St. Columba's Episcopal Church in Washington, which had a gifted preacher, and I participated in study groups. Later I taught Sunday school there with Milly's loving friend, Terry Schaefer, a TV producer. She made our sixth-graders feel cradled in affection while I tried to get them to think about who Jesus would be if he were a kid in their school. It was always disturbing to me that they invariably thought Jesus would be a "nerd." I tried to convince them that he would be a dynamic leader who would shake up the school culture as he did the world, raising up "losers" and alienating the "popular kids," probably at his own peril. Milly, too, has found momentary comfort at St. Columba's when the priests say healing prayers over her as they administer Communion. But no one has been able to restore her trust in God. "I feel abandoned by God," she says. "I feel like Job."

To help find my own answers and to help her, I asked questions of my pundit pal Fred Barnes, who is a born-again Christian. He got me reading *Mere Christianity* and other books by C. S. Lewis. And he invited me to join a newly forming men's fellowship that's become as much my "church" as St. Columba's. Members of the group and their wives pray for Milly and for me regularly, and they offer us counsel and encouragement. The group is led by Jerry Leachman, who came to be with me during Milly's surgeries. A muscular onetime University of Alabama linebacker, Jerry is an ordained minister who does not use the title "Reverend." Jerry is a freelance apostle, supported by contributions to a foundation, who spreads the message of the Lord worldwide. His "congregations" include groups of Washington politicians, businessmen, and journalists he meets with regularly, corporate and church groups he lectures to around America, and ordinary people he encounters and prays with on the street. On a visit to Russia before the fall of communism he became interested in a decrepit cancer hospital near Moscow where children were being sent to die in squalor. He adopted it as a project and has transformed it, convincing rich Americans and pharmaceutical companies to donate money and drugs. In the meantime, he has converted former Communist officials in the region around the hospital to Christianity.

Not all the members of our group are born-again, including me. Unlike Jerry and Fred, I have difficulty accepting the divinity of Jesus. I do not have a "personal relationship" with him. But I know that an ideal for humanity lies in Jesus' message and example of love, self-sacrifice, and total commitment. I am also warmed by Christianity's universal offer of redemption. As Saint Paul says, "In Christ, there is neither Jew nor Gentile, slave nor free, male nor female." And I am inspired by the description of Jesus written by the

Yale historian K. S. Latourette at the conclusion of his seven-volume study of the expansion of Christianity:

> No life ever lived on this planet has ever been so influential in
> the affairs of men. . . . From [it] has flowed a more powerful
> force for the triumphal waging of man's long battle than any
> other ever known. . . . Through it millions have been sustained
> in the greatest tragedies of life. . . . Hundreds of millions have
> been lifted from illiteracy and ignorance. . . . It has done more
> to allay the physical ills of disease and famine than any impulse
> known to man. It has emancipated millions from chattel slavery
> and millions of others from thralldom to vice. . . . It has been
> the most fruitful source of movements to lessen the horrors of
> war and to put the relations of men and nations on the basis of
> justice and peace.*

I know in my heart that, in spite of all the wrongs committed in Christ's name over the centuries, Jesus himself is a leader whose message I believe in. It's a failure on my part that I cannot yet make a full commitment of my life and soul.

For the moment I am this far along in my pilgrimage. Jerry Leachman's single favorite Bible passage—which he has insisted we memorize—is from the Old Testament: "Trust in the Lord with all your heart and lean not on your own understanding. In all ways, acknowledge Him and he will direct your path" (Proverbs 3:5). This is gradually becoming my ultimate rule for living, and it's perfect for my kind of stoicism: I will, I *must*, play the hand that's dealt me and trust in God to help me do the right thing.

* Kenneth Scott Latourette, *Advance Through the Storm*, vol. 7 of *A History of the Expansion of Christianity* (Grand Rapids, MI: Zondervan Publishing House, 1970), p. 503.

But if this works for me, what about Milly? Why was this hand, Parkinson's-plus, dealt to her? Why would the compassionate God I believe in—the creator and embodiment of power, love, beauty, and goodness in the universe—destroy her body and afflict her mind? Or permit this evil to take place? Of course, this is one of the deepest questions in theology, known as the "theodicy issue"—how to reconcile God's supposed goodness, omnipotence, and omniscience with events like the Holocaust and the suffering of innocent people from disease and disaster.

Besides being Milly's question, it's also Job's. C. S. Lewis and other sages answer the Holocaust question—not well—with the argument that God gave humans free will and we've misused it. But they have no answer for the problem of natural evil—innocent children dying of famine or cystic fibrosis, Third World villagers washed away by floods. The best I can say to Milly is that I do not think that God is punishing her for anything or that God inflicted Parkinson's upon her. I tell her that, as they say, "shit happens"— and for some reason God allows it to happen. He is also available, however, to provide comfort and instill courage. This works for me, but it does not work for her.

I do not know whether my faith would withstand my own affliction with a chronic disease. I do feel blessed that it has helped me cope with Milly's. I talk to God many times a day, mostly to ask for help for myself and strength for Milly. At various times— the first time, memorably, on an Outward Bound solo beside the Colorado River in 1994—I have asked God, "What's my purpose here?" The answer always comes back—silently, of course, but unmistakably—"Take care of Milly." I periodically have asked again, hoping some new and important mission would be added. The answer is always the same.

"Taking care of Milly" has involved, first of all, convincing her that I will be with her through any ordeal. I have done everything possible, verbally and in action, to ease the terror of abandonment so embedded by her childhood losses. That fear has largely abated, although in moments of despair Milly still tells our therapist, Dorree Lynn, that someday I will want to put her away in a nursing home or "get rid" of her. Deep down she evidently fears she will eventually become a burden too heavy for me to bear. I do all I can to convince her that I can bear it. I tell her every day, several times a day, that I love her. I kiss her good morning, every morning, the instant I awaken. She invariably is awake before I am. When I turn over she gives me a wide-eyed look of greeting. Even if it weren't our ritual, she is so adorable in such moments I couldn't help but kiss her. I regularly call her by silly names— Applesauce, Peachy Pie, Plum Pudding, Sweetpea. We share a long morning hug before I go to work that sustains me as much as I hope it does her. One capacity that Parkinson's has not impaired is Milly's ability to hug firmly. Once or twice a day I say or sing, "Have I told you lately that I love you?" Our little joke is that she always says "No," so I say it again.

On a practical level, "taking care of Milly" means providing care for her. We've spent countless hours in doctors' offices all over the country, and I've spent hours on the telephone talking to specialists, ensuring that she's had the best possible treatment. The one thing that I haven't done is try to become one of those lay experts who understands medicine so well that he or she can contribute ideas for a cure, as in the movie *Lorenzo's Oil*. I tend to trust professionals unless they prove untrustworthy, and none of Milly's doctors has ever seemed so. To the contrary, we have been fortunate to have her basic neurological care provided at NIH, the center of medical research in the United States. And through the Parkinson's Action Network I have met many of the country's other leading Parkinson's researchers, whom I've called on for advice on what advanced treatments we should consider.

We never stop looking for the right medical equipment—walkers, then wheelchairs, motorized wheelchairs, and communications devices. When we sold our house and bought our apartment, we had handrails installed along our hallways in hopes that Milly could walk from room to room. But by the time we moved in, her balance was too far gone for that to work. We also hoped that she could move around in the apartment and outside using a motorized chair, and we've bought two different models. Neither has worked. Whatever has destroyed Milly's balance also has affected her ability to "drive," causing her to run into walls and off of sidewalks.

We concluded that she would have to be pushed in a wheelchair, but that also had its problems. One chair we bought was too wide, and Milly, who lists to the right, was always hanging out of it, even when we used pillows to prop her up. Another was too narrow, and the wheels rubbed against her hip, damaging her clothes and sometimes bruising her skin. Even the chair that works best, made by Invacare, didn't come with a seatbelt. For a couple of years, if we hit a bump or were heading down the ramp into our apartment's garage, Milly might fly out of the chair and onto the ground, risking injury. This happened at least a dozen times, terrifying both of us and disturbing onlookers, until we finally figured out that we needed a belt.

When Milly first began to fall frequently and had to stop driving a car, I tried to do the housework and errand-running that she couldn't. For years we'd had a wonderful Bolivian housekeeper, Rosa Cabrera, who kept the place clean and in order. But Rosa was tiny and not strong enough to pick Milly up when she fell. She was so affected emotionally by Milly's deterioration that she stopped working for us when we moved into Washington. She visits regularly with her daughter, Jenny, our goddaughter, and Rosa cares for Milly's much-loved, very spoiled dog, whose barking at elevator noises has made her unwelcome in our condominium. Rosa remains like a member of our family, but we had to make other arrangements for daily caregiving.

Milly's friend Gloria Doyle, wheelchair-bound by a spinal tumor, for years had live-in help provided by ladies from the Philippines. Through her we found a team of indispensable and loving women who have helped Milly now for eight years. I don't believe in genetic determinism, but I do believe in cultural predisposition. Whatever it is, Philippine women seem to have a special gift for caregiving. And Grelanda Te and Felicia Relano have it bounteously, as does Nory Siwal, who spells them occasionally. They are utterly dependable, freeing me to work early or late, go out of town to make speeches, and take weekend time to get some exercise. They give Milly her shower and dress her in the morning, give her meals and medicine, take her to doctors' appointments, go to the movies with her, and try to restrain her when they go on shopping trips.

They, too, are like members of our family, and we are involved with theirs. Along with Milly's doctors and nurses at NIH, they come as our guests to Parkinson's fund-raising galas. We regularly go to Philippine weddings and anniversary celebrations. Both Grelanda and Felly retell, in a dodgy modern variation, the old-fashioned American immigrant story. Separated from her husband in the Philippines, Grelanda came to the United States on a tourist visa with the precise aim of marrying an American and escaping the limited future available to her at home. Grelanda was forty when she arrived here in 1989, but she must have looked twenty given her China-doll youthfulness now. She left four children behind with her in-laws in the town of Roxas City on the island of Visayas. Felly, a Girl Scout official unhappily married to a doctor on the island of Mindanao, won a free trip to a Scout convention in San Francisco the same year. When it was over she decided to visit a friend in Washington and then decided not to go back. She got a job as a wealthy family's housekeeper and overstayed her visa, leaving two children behind.

For a time both of them lived as illegal immigrants in a one-bedroom apartment in Maryland shared by twelve women who slept on floors and kept their belongings in paper boxes. They both eventually married Americans and became permanent legal residents. Grelanda is now a U.S. citizen; her swearing-in was an event we celebrated. For years they've worked all or part of seven days a week, sending money back to their families. Grelanda has put all of her kids through college and brought two of them to live in the United States. Both of Felly's kids now are in the United States. All of these children either are or are on their way to being high-tech professionals.

Grelanda first began working for us in 1992, while Milly was still driving and seeing clients. She virtually has become Milly's third sister. Milly counseled Grelanda on family difficulties, including a daughter-in-law's drug problems, and got me to help get her daughter, Christina, into the United States. Grelanda has watched and listened, in pain and love, as Parkinson's has diminished Milly. She comes with us every August for a week at the Longs' house in Wisconsin and sometimes on winter vacations with them to Mexico. Felly began working for us in 1998 and now is with Milly four days a week. Were it not for them, I could not make a living. I would be exhausted. And I would find it much more difficult to be patient and loving.

At night and part-time on weekends, I am Milly's caregiver.

Even with love in my heart, it is hard work, and it makes me doubly appreciate what "Milly's ladies" do. On weekdays I usually arrive home around seven-thirty. Milly has finished dinner and is sitting in her favorite green chair in our bedroom, reading and watching either the Fox News Channel or *Jeopardy* on ABC. If it's Fox, she'll have something to say about my just-concluded performance on Brit Hume's "Special Report." Fred Barnes, National Public Radio's Mara Liasson, and I debate the day's hot news with Brit on a pundit panel that concludes his show every weeknight. Milly usually lets me know that I *looked* good on the show, but that I wasn't vigorous enough in defending the Democrats against Fred's assaults from the right. She'd like me to be the down-the-line Democrat that she is but by this time knows I won't be: I'm a professional moderate, condemned (as Adlai Stevenson once mordantly said of himself) to see both sides of every question.

Our routine is that I then fix myself some dinner and eat it in the bedroom, sitting as close as I can get to Milly's chair, usually on pillows piled atop a wastebasket. If I can't make out what she is saying—as is usually the case—I ask her to take a deep breath and say just the first word. If I can't understand that, I ask for the first letter of the first word, then the second, and so on. Or I try to get her to warm up her throat by singing with me the kindergarten alphabet song and then ask her to repeat her message. Painstakingly, she tells me what she's done that day—yoga, tai chi, shopping, a movie, maybe tea with a friend—or what new project she has in mind.

I'm so inefficient, and so overcommitted, that I can never get my *Roll Call* work done at the office. So on Tuesdays and Thursdays I have to spend most of the rest of the night going through my interview notes and reading material and then writing my column. On Mondays, Wednesdays, and Fridays, though, I watch

TV with Milly while writing checks, checking e-mails, and sometimes doing laundry. When she was healthy Milly paid the bills, did most of the grocery shopping, and took clothes to the cleaners. Now I do that. In fact, I enjoy shopping because it gives me a chance to make choices that stick.

One of my favorite little joys is to go to a gourmet store and surprise Milly each week with a new type of soft cake or pie that will make her medicine easier to swallow. Key lime pie is her favorite. I also buy her Godiva chocolates or Good and Plenty candy, which she enjoys while watching TV or reading, somehow avoiding ever gaining weight. Next to her chair is a bell she rings if she wants me to quit writing, come in from the next room, and help her if she's dropped her book, can't work the channel-changer, or, most often, needs to go to the bathroom. I lift her partway out of her chair. Once she has some momentum, she can help raise herself and stand with support. After she is up, we slow-dance either to her wheelchair or all the way to the bathroom—the more exercise she gets the better—where I change her disposable underwear and then dance her back to her chair.

Before bedtime Milly always wants me to check e-mail to see whether there are messages from Alex and Andréa, the Longs, the Wheelers, or her increasing number of new pen pals. I print out what there is and either read it to her or, if she's got her glasses on, give it to her to read. She used to be intimidated by the computer and would just tell me what to e-mail back. Lately, though, she wants to write her own e-mails. So I lift her into her wheelchair and roll her to the computer. E-mailing isn't as easy as it should be for her. Even though our computer is equipped with software to aid the handicapped, it's still hard for Milly to move the cursor around the screen, click commands effectively, and hit the right keys. So I set up the e-mail program for her and let her peck out her messages. Then I correct mistakes and send the mail for her. E-mail is a great potential boon for the handicapped, but engineers need to do more to make it convenient for them.

When it's time for bed, we go back to the bathroom, where I undress Milly, put on her nightgown and new underwear, and brush her teeth. Then I roll her to the bed, open the covers, lift her, sit her down, and help her swing her legs into bed. Several years ago, when Milly developed back problems that led to surgery, we got fancy adjustable beds with head- and foot-raisers, plus massage. I never use my gadgets, but Milly does so regularly—they let her sit up and read and watch TV in bed. I'm usually dead tired by eleven-thirty or midnight, so after kissing her and telling her that I love her, I fall off to sleep quickly, holding her hand or touching her arm. She often falls asleep later, so sometimes I wake up at 5:00 A.M. and find the TV still on. I turn it off and go back to sleep. In the morning, after our kiss, I click on *Good Morning America* or *Today*. Before I get ready for work I give her the easy-to-take medicine, Sinemet and Mirapex, then take her to the bathroom once again and, if necessary, change the disposable pad on her side of the bed and give her another nightgown change.

On weekends there is more for me to do than on weekdays. Grelanda is there part of Saturdays and Sundays, but often I give Milly her breakfast, her medicine, and her shower and get her dressed. For breakfast she has a fruit-milk-juice-ice-cream drink concocted in a blender, plus a pancake or waffle soaked in syrup to make it soft. Milly cannot drink liquid from a glass. Invariably she gulps it down her windpipe. But she can usually draw it up through a straw. That is how she takes her morning drink. She gets her first doses of hard-to-take medicine with breakfast: the indispensable antidepressant Effexor, which apparently tastes awful; Amantadine, which comes in a huge red capsule that has to be emptied onto Milly's pancake; and Comtan, a giant orange tablet that has to be crushed and mixed with the pancake and syrup.

When I had saved enough money from making speeches, we had our bathroom redesigned to make it handicapped-friendly, pulling out a huge, climb-in bathtub that Milly couldn't use and replacing it with a roll-in shower enclosed in glass. I lift Milly from her wheelchair onto a shower-chair, give her a shampoo, and wash her back and face. She washes her chest. Then I ease her to a standing position and our joke is, "I'll wash the backside, you wash the front." After a rinse-off, I wrap Milly in towels, making her look like a robed Arab prince, and wheel her to brush her teeth and then put her clothes on. We have another standing joke when I help her get into her bra. I always say, as I move a breast into it, "Aha, this is the good part." And she always laughs.

On Saturday nights we go to the movies or the theater. On Sundays we often go grocery shopping together. When we take a trip I lift Milly from her wheelchair into the car, then fold up and load the chair into the trunk. At our destination I remove it and her and negotiate ramps and elevators. I am thankful for the Americans with Disabilities Act, which requires public places to be handicapped-friendly. Whenever we are in Mexico I get a sense of what America was like prior to ADA: streets are more dangerous because it takes time to get over curbs, and theaters, stores, and restaurants with stairs are all but inaccessible. When we go to the grocery together, I've figured out how to push Milly's wheelchair with one hand and drag the shopping cart with the other. This works fine except when the aisles are narrow. We've knocked over enough displays that I know which stores to avoid. On Sunday nights I cook dinner—often baked potato, which Milly finds easy to eat, but sometimes the ribs, steak, or pork chops that she loves and misses. These have to be finely chopped or ground up and mixed with potatoes for her to swallow. And then there's cleaning up to do.

I rarely resent this labor—mainly because I do not have to do it every day, all day. Always pressed for time, I get angry in traffic and yell at other drivers (with the windows up), but I do not feel enslaved by Parkinson's or sorry for myself. I do feel sorry for Milly. I do not cry often, but when I do it's when I realize how tortured she feels at being dependent and increasingly locked in her body. Were she not taking an effective antidepressant, were she sobbing daily, I would be in agony.

Without Effexor, and without Felly and Grelanda helping, both my stoicism and my Christianity would be sorely tested. My love for Milly would be tested. I think this because I finally did read Maggie Strong's book *Mainstay* and realized how lucky I am—that I am not a woman taking care of a chronically ill man, that I make enough money to hire people to help me, that my newspaper has excellent health insurance that has paid for Milly's surgery and wheelchairs without argument. And most of all, that Milly is an angel whom people always want to help. Grelanda said to me, "Sometimes we've been out and I'm tired, but Milly wants to do something else. I say, 'Milly, let's do it tomorrow.' But she looks at me with those big eyes, and I can't disappoint her, especially because she's been so loving and generous to me. So I always say, 'Okay, Milly, let's do it.' " So do I.

Other people are not so fortunate. They feel trapped, furious, oppressed, or depressed. I imagine that I would also feel that way if, for example, I were a woman whose ill husband had been forced to stop working, sharply reducing the family's income and making it impossible to hire help. I would have to work, possibly care for children, and look after my ill spouse—be on duty twenty-four hours a day, every day. If he were heavy, it might be not only exhausting to lift him but a threat to my own health. Some caregivers are required to deal with repeated life-and-death emergencies—calling ambulances, rushing to hospitals, and then waiting to see whether their loved one will be resuscitated. After years of such panics I might want my loved one not to be saved.

I know of families in which the chronically ill spouse tyrannizes the well one, constantly finding fault, making unreasonable demands, manipulating and abusing. Alzheimer's victims sometimes become violent toward their spouse. Or violent with everyone else, forcing the spouse to be constantly present. When Maggie Strong organized the Well Spouse Foundation to provide support for caregivers, she received a letter from one twenty-eight-year-old woman who summarized the facts of her life: "Husband, 31, brain tumor, unable to talk, walk or express himself, wears diapers and unable to take care of his personal hygiene; 4 children, aged 7 months to 10 years." A Florida woman described a life revolving around urine bags and concluded: "I've catheterized him, diapered him, disimpacted his bowels, carried him on my back, read for him. You name it. I'm thirty."

Strong wrote her book at a time when the plight of "well spouses" was ignored by doctors, the government, and even friends, who tended to be concerned only with the ill spouse. "The rest of the world shies away or just plain flees," she wrote. "Few people know who we are and what we need." Partly thanks to her efforts, that's changed. At least it has for me. Countless numbers of people ask, "How's Milly?" but almost as many ask, "And how are *you* doing?" They say, "I think what you're doing is great." I get special support from members of my religious fellowship and their wives. One of them, Susan Yates, the wife of the Reverend John Yates, counsels about-to-be-married couples and lectures on marriage around the country. She brought tears to my eyes by saying, "I want you to know that I use you and Milly as the model of what a marriage should be. Your love is an inspiration to everybody who knows you." One day I went to hear Fred Barnes speak to a Presbyterian church men's dinner and was stunned that half the speech was about me—"the two Morton Kondrackes, the pundit you see on television and the loving husband you don't know about."

Some people tell me, "You're a saint." I admit that for years I used to inwardly exult in that. I feigned modesty, but I was not modest. I wanted to be Saint Mort, and I wanted to be known as Saint Mort. When Milly and I go to wedding receptions, we always dance a few numbers because I know that she loved dancing and desperately misses being able to do it. But part of my motivation used to be the knowledge that people would say to one another, "Look at them. Isn't that great!" When I wheeled Milly into a room and treated her in the loving way that is normal for us, I couldn't do it without also thinking about how admirable people would think I was. I was using Milly, in effect, to secure respect from people that I feared I couldn't achieve otherwise. I do not know why I stopped doing this. In truth, I haven't entirely stopped. But one day it dawned on me that life is not for show, but for real.

A crucial moment in this phase of my pilgrimage occurred in a group therapy session led by Dorree Lynn. One of the members, a woman architect, told us that her mother, a cold and distant woman, was dying in her nineties. Only now, she said, was she able to touch her mother—and even yet, she had not hugged her. She had not hugged her for decades. This moved me. The story was a reminder of mortality and of lost opportunities. I decided that I would really try to live with all others—and not just

Milly—by a dictum that I heard in AA: "Every human contact is an opportunity." For most of my life I have viewed every human contact as a public relations challenge. Will I impress? Where will I rank? I think I now view human contact as an opportunity to connect, to help. It is a work in progress.

So far I think I have fulfilled my vow to do this one thing well—to "take care of Milly." In the process I've become a different, better person—someone I never expected to be. I have put someone else's happiness ahead of my own. And I've become dedicated to causes greater than my own advancement—those of conquering Parkinson's disease and increasing support for all disease research. I am not a saint, but I am certain that all of this is God's work. One of Milly's friends told me, "Everybody becomes a better person because of Milly." It has definitely been true for me.

6

Politics

Inside and out, the White House fairly shimmers with light at Christmastime. And so it did on December 15, 1993, when Milly and I made our first foray into politics as a way of saving her from Parkinson's disease. Each year since I covered Gerald Ford's White House in 1975 we'd been invited to one of the Christmas parties that the president and first lady host for the media and officials from the administration. The parties are so crowded that we'd stopped going regularly sometime in the 1980s. But in 1993, when Bill and Hillary Clinton were newly in office, we RSVPed immediately, hoping that we could say something to them that would accelerate Parkinson's research.

It was apparent by this time that we were falling behind in Milly's race for life. When she was first diagnosed in 1988, neurologists assured us that so much progress was being made in Parkinson's research that the disease might be cured within five or ten years. If Milly's case developed slowly, we'd hoped, there was a chance that medical science would rescue her. Over the next five years, we regularly read in newspapers and in material from Parkinson's organizations about "promising developments"—gene therapies, new surgical techniques, drug advances, and substances that might regenerate nerve tissue. But by 1993 it was becoming clear that Milly's Parkinson's was moving aggressively, and neurologists were still saying that a cure could take five or ten years, at the best.

Up to this time we had not played an active role in pushing for a cure. We had just hoped it would arrive in time. I wanted to believe that the pace of medical science was objective, not affected by outside manipulation. This assumption was contrary to everything I knew about other fields of human behavior— from the schoolyard to international relations—where people get the most they can for themselves, their friends and loved ones, and their causes. But I was still very much the Old Mort, excessively respectful of experts and intimidated by systems I didn't understand.

By the time the Clintons' Christmas invitation arrived, however, I was beginning to understand disease politics. My eyes were first opened earlier in 1993 by literature that Jill Schuker sent to us from the Parkinson's Action Network. It pointed out that Parkinson's research was deeply underfunded by the federal government in comparison to other diseases. The minute I read it, I felt that I'd let Milly down by not taking action earlier. I knew I had to do something, but I didn't know what to do. I had a twice-weekly column in *Roll Call*, a newspaper read by practically everyone on Capitol Hill, but at first it struck me that using my position to campaign for more Parkinson's money constituted unethical special pleading.

But in July of that year I decided I could write something if I disclosed my personal interest. I phoned Joan Samuelson, PAN's president, whom I hadn't yet met. On the basis of the interview, I wrote a column saying that President Clinton had given a gift of hope to victims of Parkinson's, Alzheimer's disease, diabetes, and prenatal disorders by lifting the ban that Presidents Reagan and Bush had imposed on federal funding of fetal-tissue research. But, I wrote, Clinton then "dashed that hope by cutting the funding" for research—$9 million from the budget of the National Institute of Neurological Disorders and Stroke (NINDS) and $4 million from the National Institute on Aging. I quoted Joan as saying that Parkinson's and Alzheimer's research were "sacrificial lambs to pay for cures for AIDS and cancer while trying to reduce the deficit."

Indeed, in his first budget as president in 1993 Clinton had asked for $225 million more for AIDS research, to bring the total to $1.3 billion, and $130 million more for cancer, for a total of $2.1 billion. According to what came to be known as Joan's "disparity chart," NIH then was spending an average of $1,000 a year on research to help each of the nation's 1.3 million HIV/AIDS victims. For each of 8 million cancer victims, NIH spent $260, while 4 million Alzheimer's patients got just $54 each, and 1 million Parkinson's victims $26 each. In this column I said that "a close relative of mine" had Parkinson's.

The next step in my education came just a few weeks before the White House party, at a big dinner honoring Abe Pollin, owner of Washington's pro basketball and hockey teams, whose wife, Irene, was Milly's friend and former social work colleague at the Neurology Center. The Pollins arranged for us to sit with Abe's political adviser, the Washington health lobbyist Terry Lierman, who proceeded to completely demystify medical research politics. The upshot of his tutorial was that research itself produces miracles for mankind, but getting the money for it is as dog-eat-dog as any other kind of politics.

Terry once had been staff director of the Senate Appropriations Committee. After leaving government, he became a disciple of the great medical research advocate Mary Lasker and started a firm representing disease groups and pharmaceutical companies. Terry told Milly and me that diseases were allocated research money based on the clout of their advocates—in the White House, in Congress, in the media and public opinion, and within NIH and the scientific community. Disease researchers who were receiving the most money one year had the best chance of getting more the next year, sometimes regardless of the scientific merit of their proposals. Parkinson's was bringing up the rear, he said, and probably would stay badly funded—unless the whole of NIH got a major boost in funding.

Terry also revealed to us that Bill Clinton, though he was helping AIDS and cancer research, was giving short shrift to every other disease studied at NIH, not just neurological diseases. This news stunned me, but it had credibility because Terry was a Democrat. It was news that the public was unaware of—something I could definitely write about, I said. Terry said he would put me in touch with his old friend, Senator Tom Harkin of Iowa, a champion of NIH funding who was then chairman of the appropriations subcommittee overseeing the Departments of Labor, Education, and Health and Human Services. (NIH is part of HHS.)

As luck would have it, Harkin had a hearing scheduled the very next week. A series of Nobel Prize scientists and advocates from disease groups and medical centers made the case that research funding is an investment that produces huge returns. It saves lives, reduces long-term medical costs, increases worker productivity, and provides the United States with drugs and devices it can export to the world. Yet, Harkin said, in 1993 Bill Clinton was the first U.S. president ever to submit a budget calling for a net cut in funding for NIH after inflation was taken into account. He said he anticipated that Clinton's next budget also would be "terribly inadequate."

After this hearing I wrote a column in the December 9 issue of *Roll Call* headlined "Is Medical Research an 'Investment'? Not to the Clintons." I charged that the Clinton administration was "underfunding and even discouraging medical research"— discouraging it because, as part of her newly unveiled health care reform proposal, First Lady Hillary Rodham Clinton was threatening to impose price controls on pharmaceuticals, a restriction that would undercut investment in drug research.

This column appeared after we'd received our invitation to the White House. When we arrived for the Christmas party I had no idea whether either of the Clintons had read it. It was a tough column that I hoped had gotten their attention, but I had to assume that it did not. *Roll Call* is read avidly on Capitol Hill, but only intermittently at the White House. I knew President Clinton slightly. I'd interviewed him a few times during the 1992 campaign, and I knew he watched *The McLaughlin Group*. In print and on TV, I sometimes supported him and sometimes criticized him. As a result, in a speech at one White House correspondents' dinner, he made a crack about his critics. He said he'd been called an effete intellectual by George Will, mean-spirited by Bob Novak, and "wavering and indecisive by Morton Kondracke."

Milly and I talked about the Clintons a lot. We had markedly different attitudes toward them. She revered them, believing them to be idealistic, energetic problem-solvers for whom doing good was the highest priority. In 1992 she had given $500 each to the Clinton campaign and the Democratic Party. She forgave Clinton his Gennifer Flowers scandal then and his Monica Lewinsky scandal later. I was skeptical from the outset about the integrity of both Clintons. And I became especially suspicious of Mrs. Clinton after she fired a friend of mine, the late David Ifshin, as general counsel of the Clinton 1992 election campaign. David had pushed hard for full disclosure when the Whitewater land scandal broke, whereas she wanted what amounted to a cover-up. He had warned—all too presciently—that if Clinton got elected with Whitewater still unresolved, his adversaries would secure appointment of a special prosecutor. Still, I respected President Clinton's centrist inclinations, and looking forward to the Christmas party, I believed there was a chance that the Clintons might be interested in having the conquest of a major disease as part of their legacy.

Besides glittering with light, the marble White House glows with warmth at Christmas. All the public rooms are richly decorated with trees and ornaments. As visitors arrive the Marine Band softly plays carols. No matter what political crises are brewing—this night, the murmur was that our friend Les Aspin was about to be fired as secretary of defense—it's possible to believe that peace will prevail and justice will be done, so abundantly do people seem to be possessed of goodwill.

If you attend White House Christmas parties regularly, your tree at home can be festooned with the lovely ornaments that are passed out each year as souvenirs. And if you are willing to stand in line long enough, you can put a picture of yourself and the first family on your wall. The president and his wife bravely post themselves for hours in front of a tree, shaking hands, greeting, and smiling for pictures with hundreds of guests per night over several days of parties for one group and another—media, White

House staff, campaign contributors, administration appointees, personal friends, the diplomatic corps.

As we moved slowly through the receiving line that snaked from the White House's cavernous main floor receiving room, down a stairway, and through a ground-floor hallway, Milly rehearsed what she planned to say: "Mr. President, I love the two of you. I think you're great. I tell Morton that all the time. I tell him to write nice things about you. I want to say, I have Parkinson's disease, and there isn't enough money being spent on research. I hope you'll do something about that."

She repeated the speech two or three times. I was ready to cite some figures from Joan's disparity chart and tell the Clintons that Parkinson's was a disease that could be conquered soon with an extra effort. In my mind I pictured Clinton saying, "Mort, send me some information about that." Or, "You know, we're planning next year's budget right now. I'll see what I can do. Call ——————, would you?"

When we reached the Clintons and were introduced by a military aide, Milly started, "Mr. President, I want to tell you something. I have Parkinson's disease. . . . " Then she lost track. She turned to me. "Morton, what do I want to say?"

I, even less articulate, hiked my thumb into the air and blurted: "Increase brain research." Clinton just nodded, but Mrs. Clinton chimed in, "Oh, wait till we pass health reform. We're going to do a lot!"

You move on fast in these receiving lines. That's all we got to say. I felt embarrassed that I'd been so frozen-headed. But I muttered to Milly as we walked on, "Well, you've just been lied to by the first lady of the United States."

Sadly, this was so. There was nothing in Mrs. Clinton's health care reform plan for neurological research, or much of anything at all for medical research. To make matters worse, the Clinton budget released the following February contained a mere .5 percent net increase for neurology after inflation. For NIH as a whole, Clinton requested a 4.7 percent increase, only 1.7 percent after inflation.

Mrs. Clinton compounded my cynicism with a speech at NIH in February 1994 in which she said that "for much of the last decade biomedical research has been neglected and underfunded and even unappreciated. The president intends to fix that." She claimed that the Clinton administration had provided new resources for NIH. In the previous fiscal year, she said, "the president and Congress increased the NIH budget by $631 million," and "in the face of fierce spending restraints, the president has proposed another $517 million increase for fiscal 1995."

This was artfully stated. In fact, it wasn't Clinton who produced the 1994 increase. He had called for a net cut. Congress had reversed him. And now Mrs. Clinton was claiming the credit. For the coming year, Clinton was proposing less of an increase than had been enacted for the previous year, with the lion's share going for just two favored diseases—AIDS and breast cancer.

Clinton had angered the gay rights movement, which supported him in the 1992 campaign, by failing to lift a ban on gays serving in the military, instituting the policy of "don't ask, don't tell" instead. However, in an apparent effort to mollify gays, he increased the AIDS research budget by 20 percent in his first year in office. In the meantime, women's groups were legitimately angered that breast cancer research was underfunded, and Clinton responded with a 33 percent increase in fiscal 1994 and another 28 percent the following year.

I was furious at the Clintons' overall budget levels and deceptiveness. I wrote a column citing the record, under the headline

"Clintons Promise, but Don't Deliver, on Health Research." I quoted what Mrs. Clinton had said to us at the Christmas party, identifying Milly only as "someone close to me who suffers from Parkinson's disease." This column apparently did get read at the White House. Word came back that Mrs. Clinton was furious with me. Officials said that I was being unfair to the Clintons because I didn't give them credit for the budget strategy they were pursuing—propose small increases for NIH, knowing that Congress would raise the funding, while proposing big increases for education and job training, which had a harder time in Congress. My response was that they were not offering leadership on medical research and were picking favorite diseases based on politics.

One apparent consequence of my columns was that, whereas Milly and I were rather frequently invited to White House social events during the Reagan and Bush administrations—state dinners, a Super Bowl party, tennis tournaments—we got no such invitations during the Clinton years. We even stopped being invited to Christmas parties.

After our attempt at summitry failed, we became foot soldiers—and later cavalry—in the Parkinson's advocacy movement. In 1994 we finally met Joan Samuelson, a stunning, charismatic, blond lawyer from California who had been diagnosed with Parkinson's the same year as Milly, but at the even younger age of thirty-seven. Joan had been a hiker and competitive runner. Suddenly she found that her left knee was giving out. She underwent arthroscopic surgery, but when she awakened the surgeon told her that there was nothing wrong with her knee. She burst into tears. She finally went to a neurologist, who told her she had Parkinson's.

She kept working as a lawyer until 1991, when Democrats in Congress started trying to lift the Bush administration ban on federal funding of fetal tissue research. Joan called the various

Parkinson's foundations to ask what they were doing to help. They said, in effect, "Nothing." She came to Washington on her own and started lobbying. She met up with Anne Udall, Mo's daughter, and they visited members' offices together. In 1992 a bill lifting the ban passed the House and then the Senate, with even such anti-abortion Republicans as Senators Strom Thurmond, John McCain, and Bob Dole supporting it. Dole said that lifting the ban was "the true pro-life position" in this controversy. But Bush vetoed the bill.

Joan devoted so much time to the Parkinson's cause that her marriage broke up. And she'd quit her job and used up her savings. So she and Anne Udall started the Parkinson's Action Network, raising money mainly at a Washington dinner each spring named after Mo Udall and honoring public figures who exemplified his traits—grace, public service, and humor. When Milly and I met Joan we were instantly moved by her fire and conviction. Milly and Joan have similar personalities and bonded immediately as friends and fellow Parkinson's victims. We told her we would do whatever we could to help her.

That promise has led me into activities I had never imagined I had any talent for—lobbying, political strategizing, and fundraising. Much as I stopped living mainly for my own advancement when Milly was diagnosed with Parkinson's disease, I less consciously immersed myself in a cause, a movement, when we signed on with the Parkinson's Action Network. It has become consuming. For several months of each year since then, especially since I took on chairmanship of the Udall dinner, I've spent almost as much time on Parkinson's activities as on my *Roll Call* and TV duties. In effect, I've got nearly three full-time jobs. The work has changed me for the better. In the name of conquering Parkinson's disease—and later, in the name of doubling the NIH budget—I have become bold about asking others for help, votes, and money. Working with others for these ends, I've learned what genuine fellowship is, and self-forgetting.

Joan, Milly, and I started with lobbying. For good reasons, it's against the rules for journalists to use their special access to members of Congress to lobby them, even for good causes. So at first I didn't do it, at least directly. Instead, I'd call a congressman's or senator's office, shamelessly hoping that my name, *Roll Call* connection, and *McLaughlin Group* notoriety would get us an appointment. Then Milly, Joan, and I would troop in. I would just thank the member and introduce my partners. Then Joan would make a presentation about what Parkinson's is, what it does to people, and how underfunded the research was. She'd hand around copies of her disparity chart, which almost never failed to impress. One year we passed out a chart compiled by the *Chronicle of Higher Education* estimating that NIH each year was spending $2,400 per victim on HIV/AIDS, $200 on breast cancer, $100 on prostate cancer, $78 on Alzheimer's disease, $34 on Parkinson's, and only $20 each on diabetes and coronary heart disease, the nation's most common fatal conditions. PAN's estimates were different, but made the same point.

Then she'd explain that Parkinson's was invisible on the political scene because neurologists customarily tell newly diagnosed people that Sinemet will fix their symptoms. "People don't speak out at first," she'd say, "because Sinemet does work for a while. When it doesn't and they have tremors, they want to hide. And then the day comes when they might want to speak out, but then they cannot. We are determined not to be invisible anymore." "Invisible No More" was PAN's motto.

And then Milly would tell what Parkinson's was doing to her: "I can't drive anymore," she'd say in a quavering voice. "Soon I won't be able to work. I fall and have to get stitches. I have bruises all over me. I feel dependent and worthless." Each visit she cried as she explained her plight. It was not feigned or rehearsed. It arose genuinely from her despair. Each visit Joan was moved to tears, and so were many congressional staffers. I was shaken when Milly first wept in public. In later sessions I always sat close to her to hold her hand and comfort her. At the same time we all realized—and joked about the fact in private—that Milly was getting the Parkinson's message through more effectively than anyone else. Members she met invariably remembered her later, asked about her, and wished her well. They still do.

Members of Congress are always on the lookout for compelling witnesses to appear at hearings. Joan is a regular. Milly and I have been invited to deliver testimony four times. Before the Senate Special Committee on Aging in June 1995, Milly riveted a panel chaired by Senator William Cohen. "I want to tell you," she said, "that I live in fear every day that I won't be able to talk or walk, that I'll fall, that I'll be unable to move. I fear that my face will be frozen, that I won't be able to swallow, that I'll be a living dead person like Mo Udall, who now lives like a vegetable.

"I was never sick. I was always healthy," she said. "I didn't drink or smoke or eat too much. I exercised. But now I live in fear every single day of my life. I fear that I will lose my husband, who is very nice to me and treats me wonderfully. He is very good. But I still feel that I will be a burden. I am already somewhat of a burden. I wake him up in the middle of the night to take me to the bathroom because I can't get out of bed because I'm frozen, because I can't turn.

"And then sometimes when I slide down and crawl out to the bathroom, I fall. I fall every single day," she continued. "And I am bruised all up and down my body because I can't walk sometimes.

I was in the store the other day buying sheets, and I fell. I have to have somebody with me all the time. I was really an independent person. I didn't need to have people with me. I grew up in the slums and made it and went to college and graduate school. Now suddenly I have to be dependent on people."

This hearing was called by Cohen to make the case that significantly increasing medical research funding—ideally, doubling it over a five-year period—would save the government billions of dollars in the long run by reducing the Medicare outlays required to provide care to victims of such diseases as Alzheimer's, Parkinson's, and ALS (Lou Gehrig's disease), as well as to victims of spinal cord injuries and stroke.

Milly concluded, to a hushed room of senators, aides, and spectators, "I think I am going to cost the country a lot of money because I am going to be an invalid and a good-for-nothing. I'll be no good to society. I'll be a burden on society. I don't want to be a burden."

Chairman Cohen asked me whether I had anything to add. I said, "I am here for the duration, lest you have any doubts," and I made my pitch to the committee that "everyone says that a Parkinson's cure is only five or ten years away if the money were only there." But at current budget levels, I said, NIH could fund only 10 percent of the research projects presented to it and deemed meritorious by scientific panels.

Two other witnesses at this hearing were Ben Reeve, brother of the actor Christopher Reeve, who had just suffered his devastating spinal injury, and Arthur Ullian, another spinal injury victim who became a close friend of Chris's and a close ally of mine in the cause of doubling the NIH budget.

The immediate object of Milly and Joan's lobbying was to pass the Morris K. Udall Parkinson's Research Act. The bill called for the federal government to spend $100 million a year on Parkinson's research, or $100 per victim, roughly triple the then-current amount. Many congressmen and senators said they were supportive of the bill in principle, but each time we visited an office—especially in 1995, just after Republicans took control—we'd be asked, "Where is this money going to come from?" Republicans were intent on slashing every civilian department of government. NIH was saved—and granted a small increase—only because Representative John Edward Porter of Illinois, the new chairman of the appropriations subcommittee overseeing HHS, made a special plea for the agency with House Speaker Newt Gingrich.

The NIH did not support the Udall bill. It did not like to be told by Congress in an "earmark" how much to spend on particular diseases. Rather, it wanted the power to allocate resources according to its own assessment of scientific merit. Also, the Udall bill would only *authorize* $100 million for Parkinson's. It was not an appropriation that would actually provide NIH with $100 million more to spend. That meant that, if researchers at NIH—and NINDS especially—tried to increase the Parkinson's effort, they would have to rob money from some other disease research. As part of its effort to stymie the bill, NIH regularly disputed PAN's numbers, claiming for a time (but no longer) that fewer than one million Americans suffered from Parkinson's and that NIH then was devoting more than $60 million to researching it. This is a dispute that goes on and on.

More than one conservative Republican we visited looked at Joan's disparity chart, expressed sympathy with our cause, and declared, "We can get the money for Parkinson's from AIDS." A few members added, "Preventable disease," referring to AIDS. I confess, I did not argue with them. When word got around in the disease community that we were using the chart—the American

Heart Association had a similar one—the gay rights movement reacted angrily. Gary Rose, spokesman for the AIDS Action Council, was quoted in the *National Journal* as saying that the Parkinson's Action Network was "AIDS-phobic"—implying, of course, homophobic. In fact, Joan Samuelson, a liberal Democrat to the core, had no anti-gay inclinations whatsoever. She just wanted more money for Parkinson's. Moreover, the Udall bill said nothing about where a money boost for Parkinson's would come from.

For four years a newly energized Parkinson's community rallied around the Udall bill. Much of the time the various groups making up the community—chiefly the American Parkinson's Disease Association (APDA), made up of patient support groups around the nation; the National Parkinson's Foundation (NPF), a research foundation; and PAN—regarded each other as competitors for contributions and preeminence. At one point the NPF cut off its support for PAN and hired its own Washington lobbyist, who proceeded to do whatever he could to undercut Joan, even with members of Congress. One of the original sponsors of the Udall bill, Senator Mark Hatfield, threatened to stop pushing it if the groups didn't stop squabbling. Ultimately they did stop and instead joined in bombarding members of Congress with letters and visits from Parkinson's sufferers around the country.

One celebrated effort was mounted by the Tucson real estate investor Bob Dolezal to get Arizona's senior senator, John McCain, to support the bill. Diagnosed in November 1992, Dolezal first wrote to McCain in 1993. He got back a form letter thanking him for his views. He shifted his attention to Representative James Kolbe and gained his support rather easily. Then he turned back to McCain. His mail and phone calls started getting answered—impatiently—by a particular McCain aide. Dolezal bombarded him with correspondence designed to prove that NIH was overstating its Parkinson's budget and asking McCain to investigate. The aide kept responding in language indicating that he believed what NIH was saying.

Finally, in March 1996, Dolezal exploded in an e-mail that ended: "One can reach one of three conclusions: The NIH is stonewalling and doesn't want the data made public; that the request of the senior senator from Arizona has been cavalierly disdained by NIH; or that the senior senator from Arizona never seriously pursued this matter, and really doesn't give a damn. Which one gets your vote?" This outburst had consequences, short- and long-term. Somehow word got back to the University of Arizona, which promptly severed connections (since restored) with the Tucson chapter of APDA, which Dolezal headed. That response not only inspired Dolezal to launch a statewide campaign in Arizona's Parkinson's community to work on McCain but convinced him to fly to Washington to visit McCain personally.

He took along Brad Udall, Mo's younger son and look-alike, who was a board member of PAN, and MaryHelen Davila, a Parkinson's activist and sufferer from Phoenix. When they got to McCain's office they were greeted by two aides who were getting ready to say that McCain was sorry but he couldn't sign on to the bill. Mrs. Davila was close to tears. Suddenly a door opened, and McCain walked in. "Boy, do you look like your father," he said to Udall. Mrs. Davila told McCain what Parkinson's was doing to her—and cried. Dolezal launched into the Parkinson's case. McCain interjected that he did not like to earmark for specific diseases. Dolezal kept spouting statistics and arguments.

Suddenly McCain put up his hand. "Okay, that's enough. I'll co-sponsor the bill." This time Dolezal began crying. "It was one of the greatest experiences of my life," he told me.

When Mark Hatfield retired in 1997 after thirty years in the Senate, it became crucial for the Parkinson's movement to find an influential Republican to carry the cause. In the House the co-sponsors were Republican Representative Fred Upton of Michigan and Democrat Henry Waxman of California. In the Senate, Paul Wellstone of Minnesota, both of whose parents had died with Parkinson's, was our lead Democrat. In January 1997, Dolezal wrote to McCain, suggesting that it would be especially appropriate for him to take the lead given his friendship with Mo Udall. Within a week Dolezal got a call from McCain's office with the word: the senator would do it. "I let out a whoop and a holler," Dolezal told me. The first person he called with the news was Joan Samuelson.

On September 3, 1997, McCain and Wellstone offered the measure as a floor amendment to the annual appropriation for the Departments of Labor, Education, and Health and Human Services. Thanks to the Parkinson's groups' joint lobbying efforts, it had sixty-seven co-sponsors. There was a brief floor debate in which McCain said that "there is a gross inequity here that needs rectification," citing figures from Joan's disparity chart. The vote to approve the Udall bill was overwhelming, 95–3. However, the Senate fight was not yet over. The next day, pro-life Senators Dan Coats of Indiana and Don Nickles of Oklahoma planned to amend the Udall bill with language reviving the Reagan-Bush ban on federal funding for fetal tissue research. Joan and PAN's policy coordinator, Mike Claeys, were at PAN's office in Santa Rosa, California, and from there spent all night soliciting statements from scientists on the importance of the research and faxing material to friendly senators in Washington. The next day the Coats-Nickles amendment was defeated, 60–38. The Parkinson's movement had achieved an astounding victory.

In the House of Representatives, though, we had problems. First, whenever the right-to-life movement heard the word "Parkinson's," it immediately thought "abortion" and started gearing up to attach an amendment reviving the fetal-tissue ban. The right-to-lifers' logic is that any benefit derived from abortions— even saving lives—lightens its stigma and encourages more abortions. In 1997 the pro-life movement had not yet focused its energies on banning partial-birth abortions, so fetal-tissue research was vulnerable politically. I went to see aides to Speaker Gingrich, for example, to see whether he would help on the Udall bill. The word came back: "Can't do it. The right-to-lifers won't like it."

Our second problem in the House lay with Representative Porter. Though he was a hero in the cause of medical research, Porter, backing up NIH Director Dr. Harold Varmus, was death on disease earmarking. Porter said that he opposed "politicizing" disease research and trusted the judgment of NIH scientists to set priorities. In various conversations we had over the years, he readily acknowledged that history was replete with examples of congressional or White House intervention on behalf of AIDS, cancer, and other diseases. But he was determined not to let the pattern spread. The Parkinson's movement definitely wanted an earmark if it could get one. He was determined to stop it.

I went to Porter and said, "The Senate is putting the Udall bill into the appropriation. Will you agree not to fight it?" After all, I said, the bill really was not an earmark since it merely *authorized* NIH to spend $100 million. It didn't appropriate the money or command NIH to spend it. To my combined amazement and trepidation, he said, "Okay, if you can get the authorizers not to oppose it. You've got to talk to them." The "authorizers" were the leading Republicans on the House Commerce Committee and its health subcommittee, staunch right-to-lifers. I think Porter may have doubted that we would ever be able to get their assent.

I went to see two of them. Both, to my further amazement and gratification, said they would look the other way. One of them, whose office Milly, Joan, and I had visited, not only agreed to raise no objection but volunteered to go to Porter and tell him his position—provided I breathed not a word about it. Out of gratitude, I'm still protecting his secret. The other, Representative Tom Bliley of Virginia, then chairman of the House Commerce Committee, also talked to Porter and incurred the wrath of fellow anti-abortionists when they learned what he'd done. With Porter keeping his word, the Udall bill survived a House-Senate conference on the Labor-HHS appropriation. Its passage was hailed among Parkinson's victims and advocates around the country as a moment of triumph. Indeed, we were invisible no more.

On November 13, 1997, President Clinton held a ceremony in the East Room to commemorate the appropriations bill becoming law. Clinton's priority in the measure was major new education funding, and that was the focus of the event. But he did invite Mo Udall's wife, Norma, to stand on the podium with him. Clinton had said on a number of other occasions over the years, "We're going to lick Parkinson's disease," but this time he mentioned the disease only in passing.

Though this was a moment of celebration, the old intra-Parkinson's rivalry reemerged. Because Norma Udall was on the National Parkinson's Foundation board, the White House asked NPF for a list of persons to invite to the ceremony. The NPF, in keeping with its competitive attitude toward other Parkinson's groups, furnished only the names of its own leaders. Fortunately, Joan found out about the ploy and called a friend at the White House, who got Joan, Milly, me, and the APDA's Washington representative invited, too. At the event I could not resist walking up to the NPF group and saying, "You guys make me sick." The NPF later changed its management and became more collegial.

Though it was a tremendous victory, passage of the Udall bill did not guarantee that one cent more would be spent on Parkinson's research. Even though it passed as an amendment to an appropriations bill, the Udall bill was not an appropriation. Actually getting $100 million spent directly on Parkinson's remains to this day the prime task of the Parkinson's movement, in spite of testimony from scientist after scientist that this disease is conquerable.

Where should the money come from? My first instinct—based partly on my knowledge of the funding disparities, and partly perhaps on prejudice—was to take it away from HIV/AIDS. It struck me as deeply unfair that the government was spending something like seventy times the amount per victim on AIDS as on the disease that was killing my wife. And my wife was blameless in her predicament. AIDS victims, in the main, got their disease by indulging in unprotected and often promiscuous sex and by injecting drugs with dirty needles. My attitude changed, but I cannot deny that I harbored it for a time.

In 1996 I began working on a PBS documentary, "The Politics of Medicine," which ran on the network in April 1997. It was part of a documentary series, *National Desk*, that Fred Barnes and I started along with the Hollywood screenwriter Lionel Chetwynd. In doing research for the show, I found government data showing that during the first three years of the Clinton administration the research budget for AIDS had increased 40 percent, the prevention budget 24 percent, the treatment budget 176 percent, and overall spending on AIDS 77 percent. Meanwhile, despite occasional nice words from the president, Parkinson's spending was flat.

One of the first people I interviewed on camera for the show was the AIDS activist (and victim) Gary Rose, who had attacked PAN over the disparity chart. When I asked him about that, he accused me and PAN of telling Congress that the plight of AIDS victims was "their own fault, so give the money to us." He said, "After watching hundreds of my friends die, I find that argument repulsive. To put the blame on the victim, whether it's HIV or lung cancer, is immoral.

"Most people don't have a choice about getting HIV-infected," he said. "I didn't have a choice. To say to someone, 'You should have worn a condom,' just think about that: if HIV were a disease primarily of white, middle-aged heterosexual men, who'd tell them, 'You have to wear a condom for the rest of your life'? It wouldn't happen. Human beings like to have sex, and they like it to be natural and not negotiated."

As I sat across from him, I felt myself getting furious at the implication of his argument: that research into Parkinson's was being starved so that gay men could have "unnegotiated" sex. I burst out at him: "Well, as a citizen and as somebody who's married to someone who has Parkinson's, the way I look at it is, the AIDS community has a preventable disease. It has mobilized itself very carefully, using Hollywood and the gay community, has impacted Congress, has gotten an enormous amount of money spent on it. As a consequence, the disease research that I care about is underfunded. Why am I wrong?"

He burst back, "Who are we? Homosexuals, drug addicts, poor black people. Hollywood came with us only after we began to die. If the most condemned sections of American society can pull together and do the remarkable and miraculous thing that we've done. . . . We started without any power, without money. We had nothing. We had *nada*. No one would talk to us. If we can build out of those garbagy tools, I don't know how anybody in good faith can come after us and say, 'You really don't deserve your success.'

"I'm just incredibly offended at being condemned for success that has cost me every person I cared about in my entire life. This epidemic has decimated my entire peer group. Everybody that I've worked with, cared about, lived with. And out of that pain, we've developed a movement, a process where we could cure this disease in ten years. And then to have somebody coming after me and saying, 'You don't deserve that. Give some of it to us'? I'm sorry, I don't think that's moral."

He finished me off with a challenge: "Are *you* going to stop working on television and become a full-time Parkinson's advocate? When you've done that, when thousands of other people have done that for Parkinson's, when you have given up your lives to find a cure, then you come back to me and say, 'Give up some of yours.'"

It was a powerful rebuttal, but Rose made an even stronger argument that decisively convinced me that there was no future in trying to rob AIDS to help Parkinson's: "Even if the money were cut from AIDS research," he said, "it wouldn't go to Parkinson's. It would go to the next most powerful disease." He cited breast cancer research, which was being pushed by a powerful coalition of women's groups and the White House, and diabetes, at the time the favored disease of Republicans because Speaker Gingrich's then-mother-in-law suffered from it. I knew instantly that Rose was completely correct and that the funding definitely had to come from somewhere else.

There were two good ways to go. The one that I chose—manically for a time—was to campaign for doubling the NIH budget in hopes that the rising tide would lift the Parkinson's boat. The route that Joan concentrated on—with me helping by giving advice, lobbying, and raising money—was for the Parkinson's movement to emulate the AIDS movement rather than fight it. That meant organizing the Parkinson's community, creating a fuss, gaining visibility, finding a star spokesperson, and lobbying tirelessly with Congress and the White House. Just as the AIDS movement has most of the entertainment industry wearing red ribbons and breast cancer has people wearing pink ones, the Parkinson's movement now has a button like the international no-parking symbol, with a red slash over the letters PD.

Just as AIDS has Elizabeth Taylor as a spokeswoman, juvenile diabetes has Mary Tyler Moore, and breast cancer has Tipper Gore, who also advocates for mental illness, Joan tried to enlist a prominent Parkinson's victim to speak for us. Prior to Michael J. Fox's announcement in late 1998 that he had Parkinson's, the most visible victims of the disease were Attorney General Janet Reno, who declined to be involved in disease advocacy, and Muhammad Ali. The Champ did appear before Congress on behalf of increased research, but the disease has rendered him unable to speak.

The object of the Parkinson's movement's post-Udall lobbying was to get Congress to actually appropriate $100 million for Parkinson's research—or to write language as close to a directive earmark as we could persuade Porter and other congressional leaders to accept. Other diseases kept getting them. One year Gingrich and former White House Chief of Staff Erskine Bowles, whose child suffers from juvenile diabetes, quietly put an extra $300 million for diabetes research into a final budget agreement. Another year Senator Ted Stevens, chairman of the Senate Appropriations Committee, became irritated that prostate cancer was getting less attention than breast cancer and added $50 million for that. In truth, Parkinson's also benefited from inside action when former Republican Representative Joe McDade, a member of the House Appropriations Committee, was diagnosed with Parkinson's in 1996 and created a $25 million fund for neurotoxin research in the Defense Department.

In 1998, in an effort to get a $100 million earmark for Parkinson's in the NIH budget, I went with Joan to talk to the Udall bill's co-sponsor, Senator John McCain, whom I admired—along with the bulk of the Washington press corps—for his heroism, frankness, independence, and availability. I also admired him for his friendship with and loyalty to Mo Udall. I'd written columns comparing McCain to Theodore Roosevelt and urging him to run for president in 2000. But the encounter over Parkinson's convinced me that—noble soul though he is—McCain was not White House material after all.

We met McCain in an ornate room just off the Senate floor. He listened as we explained that NIH, despite the Udall bill, was refusing to significantly increase Parkinson's funding and probably would not do so without a command from Congress. Would he co-sponsor a floor amendment with Wellstone to write $100 million into the Labor-HHS appropriations bill? McCain became irate. "This is earmarking," he said. "This is pork. I have spent my entire congressional career fighting this sort of thing. If you're looking for somebody to do this, I'm not your guy."

I was taken aback and asked, "If you believed that the United States military needed a certain weapon to protect the nation's security, but the appropriations committee refused to fund it, you wouldn't fight on the Senate floor to get the money?"

"That's right," he said. "That's pork. I would never do it." I decided then that McCain, despite his virtues, was simply too rigid to be a good president. Somebody else, I thought, had to represent a golden mean between the slippery flexibility of Bill Clinton and McCain's refusal to bend on one principle for the sake of a worthier one. In 2000, McCain became a further disappointment. Running for the Republican nomination, McCain was attacked by right-to-lifers backing George W. Bush for his past support of fetal-tissue research. He defended that position, but came out against federal funding of highly promising research using stem cells derived from leftover embryos at fertilization clinics.

Still, McCain is a hero to the Parkinson's movement for sponsoring the Udall bill in the beginning, as well as for helping PAN raise money. In 1999 we asked him to accept a Udall Award at PAN's annual dinner. I had taken over chairmanship of the dinner in 1997 and, by enlisting every friend Milly and I had and calling on corporate lobbyists, had increased the dinner's income from $91,000 to $222,000. In 1998 we brought in $375,000, partly because David Bradley, a member of Jerry Leachman's religious fellowship, and his wife, Katherine, pledged $50,000 a year for three years. In 1999 another friend, Kathy Kemper, told guests at one of her speaker breakfasts about Milly's plight. On the spot, the Washington entrepreneur Jon Ledecky pledged $25,000 in the first of many demonstrations of his generosity. That year the indispensable event planner for the dinner, Renee Gardner, suggested that we ask McCain whether, as honoree, he could help us raise money. He put his fund-raising juggernaut into a practice round for the upcoming 2000 campaign. Dozens of companies doing business before his Senate Commerce Committee—telecommunications firms, airlines, power companies—bought tables. We reached $510,000. In 2000, when we honored Representative Porter and Senator Connie Mack of Florida, who were retiring from Congress, we raised $721,000. Of course, that year Michael J. Fox was our star.

Every year, besides raising money, these dinners are a joy, one of the rare big Washington dinners that people leave feeling warm and happy. It's mainly because members of the Udall family—Anne and Mo Udall's other kids, Mark (now a congressman from Colorado), Brad, and Kate—hilariously riff on each other, showing they have inherited Mo's gene for humor. It's also because Joan Samuelson annually gives a moving speech about the plight of Parkinson's patients and the hope we have for a cure. Every year I get credited with pulling off another financial miracle, and I thank those who really make it possible. And every year speakers give special tribute to Milly as one of the heroines of the Parkinson's movement. Every year the tributes have increasing poignancy. The cure is not in hand. The money to find the cure is still not being spent. And Milly's time is running out.

7

God's Work

On January 31, 2000, the day before George W. Bush lost the New Hampshire primary to John McCain, I slipped into a makeup room at Manchester TV station WMUR, where Bush was cleaning his face after a Fox News appearance. He knew who I was because I'd interviewed him for a profile in *Reader's Digest* the year before. I said, "Can I write you a letter about my favorite cause?"

I got rattled—first, because I feared, as usual, that I wouldn't deliver my pitch well to a possible future president. And second, because I was afraid that my news colleagues would overhear me and think I was using my commentator's access for lobbying. Which, of course, is exactly what I was doing.

"What cause is that?" he asked.

"Doubling the NIH budget," I started. "It's . . . "

"I'm for it," he said. "I've talked to Connie Mack about it. I told him I'm for it. It's the right thing to do."

Actually, I already knew that Senator Mack had talked to Bush.

And I'd heard that Bush had responded favorably. For months I'd been lobbying various Bush advisers and had urged one of them to ask Mack to call Bush. But I wanted to hear it for myself from the candidate and to put in a special pitch for brain research, especially for Parkinson's.

So I said, just as inarticulately as I'd done at the Clintons' Christmas party, "Think brains."

"Brain cancer?" he asked.

"No, neurology," I said. I made a botch of my speech. "Great things are happening," I said. "Neurodegenerative factors. . . . No, I mean, something called neural growth factors. . . . Great implications for Alzheimer's, ALS, stroke, Parkinson's. Great things are happening. . . ."

I do know how to be articulate about this. Just a few days before, when Michael J. Fox announced he would be leaving his show, *Spin City*, to work for a Parkinson's cure, I had appeared on NBC's *Today Show* and delivered a flawless, on-message case for more Parkinson's funding. But I muffed this encounter with Bush. I still could not ask the highest-level big shots for help with something I care desperately about. It was neurotic.

I did finish with my favorite political argument for Republicans: "Republicans in Congress have been increasing NIH by 15 percent a year, ramping up to double. They never take credit for it."

"They don't know what they are doing," Bush said.

"Al Gore only wants to double the cancer budget, not the whole," I volunteered, hoping he'd try to trump Gore and make doubling the NIH budget a centerpiece of his campaign.

"No," Bush said, "I'm for doubling the whole—what, over ten years?"

"No," I said, "five. They can do it over five. NIH can absorb it over five."

"Okay, I'm for it."

If President Bush delivers on his promise, this two-minute encounter—tongue-tangled though I was—may go down as a high point in my involvement in the noble campaign to get the U.S. government to provide scientists with money to do more of the medical research necessary to cure diseases. For me, this started as and remains a strategy to increase Parkinson's funding. But it's also a cause I believe in profoundly on its own. I consider it God's work.

I joined up part-time right after Milly and I met Terry Lierman in 1993, when I started writing columns criticizing Clinton's budgets and publicizing the efforts of research advocates like Senators Harkin and Hatfield. For several years they had been urging Congress to create a special trust fund for medical research, financed with a 1 percent tax on health insurance premiums. The idea was torpedoed by the insurance industry and by Republicans in Congress, so the fight to increase NIH funding still has to be fought year by year through the standard appropriations process. Lifesaving research has to compete, first, with defense, highways, national parks, law enforcement, and all the other functions of government. Then, because of the way the congressional budget process works, it has to compete with other humanitarian programs—education, job training, worker safety, and public health delivery.

When Milly and I lobbied with Joan Samuelson for more Parkinson's money, members of Congress kept asking us in effect, "Whose lifeline shall we cut to throw one to you?" Even before Gary Rose convinced me it was wrong—on many levels—to cut

AIDS, I decided that doubling NIH was the cause I would work on. The main message of my PBS documentary in the spring of 1997 was that, without more NIH money, all disease groups (and victims) inevitably would continue to be pitted against each other in a cruel, zero-sum competition for resources, with the most politically powerful getting the most. The beneficial flip side could be that, with more money, all could benefit. And a breakthrough in one area of research—say, diabetes—could produce progress in other areas, like AIDS, cancer, and vascular diseases.

At the time the documentary ran, the nation was spending $37 billion on medical research. Of this, the federal government accounted for $14 billion, $12 billion through NIH. NIH concentrates on basic research—on cell functions and the molecules and genes that cause and might cure disease—and does some so-called translational research to convert these discoveries into actual cures. NIH distributes 90 percent of its money to university researchers, who compete for grants now averaging $275,000 per year. The other 10 percent finances research at the NIH complex in Bethesda, Maryland. Drug and biomedical companies were spending about $19 billion in 1997, some on basic research but most on the development of medicines and devices that would make a profit. Independent research institutions contributed another $4 billion. My show made the point that medical research was deeply underfunded, representing less than 4 percent of the nation's overall health outlays every year. Meanwhile, 10 percent of defense spending went for research. In the computer industry, research represented 15 percent of revenues.

Doubling NIH from $12 billion to $24 billion would involve a cumulative five-year spending increase of about $30 billion—a pittance in comparison to the $270 billion annual defense budget or total U.S. health spending of $1 trillion a year. A subsequent congressional study estimated that the nation spends $1.3 trillion each year paying the direct medical costs of treating disease. "Indirect" costs, including reduced ability to work, amount to another $1.7 trillion.

Thanks to the show's producer, the screenwriter Lionel Chetwynd, "The Politics of Medicine" put faces and life stories on various diseases and groups. Joan and Milly represented Parkinson's. Arthur Ullian and Chris Reeve talked about spinal cord injury, with Chris expressing the hope that he might walk again. Senator Mack and Fran Visco of the National Breast Cancer Coalition described their battles with cancer. Gary Rose represented AIDS. The documentary got a lot of favorable comment from disease groups around the country and helped cement lasting alliances with Arthur Ullian, Tom Harkin, and Connie Mack, three of the nation's most indefatigable campaigners for medical research.

Ullian, a successful Boston real estate developer, sustained his spinal injury in 1991. He was riding a bicycle down a country road when the front wheel hit a stone and he was thrown forward. He was wearing a helmet, but his chin hit the pavement. The fall left him wheelchair-bound, unable to walk and impaired in his ability to use his arms and hands. He had been a violin player since childhood and was a member of a chamber orchestra. "I had a tremendous amount of denial," he said. "I thought maybe I would be able to play it again. But in the end I had to sell it."

Arthur is a charming, clear-thinking, eloquent man of indomitable will. The combination makes him enormously effective as an activist. He will call anyone—politician, medical school dean, business tycoon, journalist—to make his case. After his accident he first affiliated with and then became president of the National Council on Spinal Cord Injury. Then he realized, following the same logic as mine, that increased research on spinal injuries depended upon increased neurological research. So he founded END, the National Campaign to End Neurological Diseases. And then he realized that increased neuroscience funding depended on overall research increases, and he helped form the Task Force on Health Care and the Economy.

Arthur's committee has enlisted such experts as the financial guru Peter Lynch and various biomedical and computer executives to make the case to Congress, the White House, and the Federal Reserve that the Medicare system can be saved from bankruptcy by postponing the onset of chronic disease through research. Delaying the onset of Alzheimer's by five years, for instance, could save $50 billion a year. Curing Parkinson's could save about $25 billion. Ullian's group also argues that the long-run health of the U.S. economy depends upon high-tech research that will produce pharmaceuticals, gene therapies, computer software, and medical devices that American companies can sell to the world. I've used Arthur's studies and congressional testimony as the basis for many newspaper columns and speeches.

Connie Mack, meanwhile, became a crusader because his family has been cursed with cancer. His younger brother, Michael, developed melanoma on his scalp in his twenties and died, with Connie sitting at his bedside, after years of chemotherapy, radiation, and surgery. Connie himself developed melanoma, but it was caught before it spread. His wife Priscilla is a breast cancer survivor and a key executive in the "Race for a Cure" movement. Connie's father, son of the legendary baseball great, died of pancreatic cancer. Thankfully, Senator Mack became an advocate, not for a narrowly focused "war on cancer," but for a broad-front campaign against all disease. I liked Mack so much that I wrote columns both in 1996 and 2000 urging that he be picked as the Republican vice presidential candidate. In 1996 he nearly was, and Bob Dole said afterward that he wished he had picked Connie. In 2000 Mack's selection might have prevented George W. Bush's near-loss to Al Gore in Florida.

Arthur, Terry Lierman, and Connie Mack are only a few of the noble souls I've encountered in the movement to double the NIH budget. Senator Harkin became an advocate because he has a deaf brother and has lost close relatives to cancer. Former Congressman Porter had no personal or family affliction but became a champion after attending so-called public witness hearings each year before the Labor-HHS appropriations subcommittee. These sessions have been dubbed "Mother Theresa's waiting room" because all those testifying have wrenching, meritorious pleas to make. A stiff-seeming Presbyterian from the tony northern suburbs of Chicago, Porter says he was especially moved by a fifty-year-old woman who appeared with her husband, fifty-four, a former Navy flier in Vietnam and test pilot, who had Alzheimer's disease. "Now the love of my life doesn't even know me," the woman testified. "I will be caring for him for the next twenty-five years, but he won't know who I am."

In 1995 Porter saved NIH from the draconian budget cuts his fellow Republicans were imposing on all domestic programs. In the frenetic first hundred days of the Newt Gingrich era, the House passed a budget resolution calling for a 25 percent cut in NIH funding over five years. Just installed as chairman of the Labor-HHS subcommittee, Porter organized a group of biomedical CEOs and Nobel laureates to meet with Gingrich. They gathered in Gingrich's "dinosaur room," where the new speaker, a zoology fan, had huge bones on display. Gingrich started out the meeting saying, "There isn't a program in the U.S. government that can't be cut by 5 percent a year." On the contrary, the scientists and CEOs said, NIH cuts would be catastrophic for university research and would have negative ripple effects on pharmaceutical and biotech industries and the U.S. economy.

By the end of the meeting Gingrich had promised to reconsider the cuts and even showed his visitors a book chapter he had written on the key role that technology would play in America's future. Meanwhile, Hatfield, chairman of the Senate Appropriations Committee, conducted a similar campaign on his side of Capitol Hill. The Senate budget resolution originally called for a 50 percent cut in NIH over five years. Porter and Hatfield convinced their colleagues that NIH should be exempted from budget slashing. In fact, they won a 5.8 percent increase for fiscal year 1996.

In previous years there had been no regular pattern to NIH funding. During fiscal year 1993, the last year of Bush's father's administration, the Democratic Congress voted an increase of 15.6 percent. During Clinton's first year, fiscal year 1994, the increase was 5.9 percent. And in 1995, the year before Republicans took over, it was just 3.6 percent. To double NIH over five years would take annual increases of 15 percent. The movement was a long way from that.

At first, my main activity was to boost doubling in *Roll Call* columns. I used every possible news peg I could find. After Christopher Reeve delivered a riveting appeal at the Democratic National Convention in August 1996 for the nation to launch a crusade against disease similar to Franklin Roosevelt's campaign against poverty and despair during the Great Depression, I wrote a column supporting him. But I also warned that Reeve was being used by President Clinton. That May, I noted, Chris had visited the White House. On the spot, Clinton had promised $10 million more for spinal cord research, a 25 percent increase. The money never materialized, however.

Terry Lierman and two associates in his lobbying firm, Ed Long and Marguerite Donoghue, always had advance word on congressional and White House budget machinations, and this information provided grist for many columns. In December 1996, for instance, they tipped me that Clinton's budget office was calling for a $200 million cut in NIH funding for the next fiscal year. This caused an uproar among NIH supporters. Porter called it "unacceptable." The following February, Clinton actually proposed a 4.0 percent increase—still barely enough to keep up with inflation. Mack persuaded fellow Senate Republicans to put the doubling of NIH funding on their agenda for the 105th Congress, but it was ranked only item number 11. When Mack, Harkin, and Pennsylvania's Arlen Specter offered a floor amendment proposing to increase NIH by $1 billion, or 7.5 percent, the Clinton administration opposed it. The bill failed, 63–37. Porter said, after Clinton announced a "national goal" of finding an AIDS vaccine in ten years, that Clinton "is very good at rhetoric, but there's been no leadership when it comes to substance or resources." Ultimately that year the good guys did push a 6.8 percent increase through Congress. The next fiscal year, 1998, Clinton's budget called for just a 2.6 percent NIH increase. Congress approved 7.1 percent. In fiscal 1999, Clinton called for an 8.0 percent increase. Congress raised the mark to 14.3 percent.

In his 1999 State of the Union message, Clinton said that "thanks to bipartisan support for medical research, we are on the verge of new treatments to prevent or delay diseases from

Parkinson's to Alzheimer's, from arthritis to cancer." People called me up afterward and said, "Hey, did you hear? The president mentioned Parkinson's!" I wrote a column saying that I was grateful, but asking where the money was. Indeed, when Clinton's fiscal 2000 budget came out the following month, it proposed only 2.0 percent more for medical research.

Even though I criticized Clinton a lot for lowballing medical research, I still had hopes for him. "Clinton's golden opportunity to make a place in history lies in backing—and leading—a bipartisan effort to double the NIH budget," I wrote in one column. In fact, it became one of my favorite themes that "championing major increases in biomedical research offers a magnificent legacy to President Clinton or a Member of Congress: for the next 50 years, he or she would share in the credit every time a disease is conquered." Moreover, I argued repeatedly—as I had meant to with Bush in the TV studio—that politicians who pushed for doubling NIH funding "could derive political credit from every citizen who faces the fear of a dreaded disease." One initiative Clinton did take was to more than triple funding for the National Human Genome Project, which may lead to strategic disease-fighting discoveries.

Besides writing columns, I got involved in the cause even more deeply in 1996. I was on a plane with my friend Paul Johnson, head of the Washington office of Fleishman Hillard, one of the world's largest public relations firms. Paul's wife, Lisa, once had been Milly's exercise therapist. I told him the dilemma: medical research is a great cause and no one's against it, but it has no political priority, no oomph. Some years Congress increases the budget by 7 percent, but the next year it's threatened with cuts. I said it would be great if somebody could organize disease victims and activists in each congressional district to lobby members and maybe round up a planeload of Hollywood stars with disease connections to descend on Washington for a high-visibility lobbying blitz.

Paul said, "Hey, let's start an organization." Thus was born America's Campaign for Medical Breakthroughs, informally known as NIH2. For two years it became my obsession. Paul Johnson thought we could raise $1 million or even $2 million a year from pharmaceutical companies and organize at the grass roots, create a web site, commission polls, get advertising companies to write public service ads for newspapers and TV, convince health writers to mention NIH funding when they wrote "new discovery" stories, and do inside-the-Beltway lobbying.

I called up other friends to join the core group: Terry Lierman; the super-lobbyist Ken Duberstein, who'd been White House chief of staff under Ronald Reagan; and Peter Teeley, Washington representative of the biotech firm Amgen, who volunteered to help raise pharmaceutical money. Arthur Ullian also became a member. Paul had aides at Fleishman Hillard draw up an elaborate strategic plan. Connie Mack and Tom Harkin agreed to vouch for us with the drug companies.

The truth is that, despite frenetic efforts, NIH2 had little to do with subsequent increases in NIH funding. Others deserve the credit. We ultimately raised only $250,000 and, with that, created more motion than progress. I spent a good deal of time trying to convince another advocacy group that we were not out to steal its funding and mission. Our cause was worthy, but some of our initiatives turned into low comedy. In March 1998, Chris Reeve generously agreed to come to Washington to accept a Udall Award at PAN's dinner and to appear at an NIH2 press conference the next day on Capitol Hill. For Reeve, who breathes through a respirator, any travel is life-threatening, so his appearances were heroic and stellar. He and Mary Tyler Moore attracted a big crowd of reporters and members of Congress. But the event turned into a misadventure.

As master of ceremonies for the event, I skillfully navigated the problem of who should speak first by letting our congressional angels, Harkin and Mack, choose between themselves. Then, as they were making their opening remarks, Senator Edward Kennedy tugged at my sleeve. Citing a pressing appointment, he asked to speak next. I assented. The second I introduced him, there was commotion. Senator Arlen Specter, chairman of the Senate appropriations subcommittee overseeing NIH, walked out in a huff. His subcommittee aide actually grabbed Marguerite Donoghue around the throat and hissed, "Senator Kennedy! Is *he* the chairman?" After the press conference I was inundated with phone calls warning me that Specter was furious at the slight. I promptly composed an abject, obsequious apology letter and hand-delivered it to his office. I got no reply. Senator Specter, though stalwart on behalf of medical research, is a notoriously difficult man.

The NIH2 core group persisted in trying to advance the cause. We heard that Health and Human Services Secretary Donna Shalala was promoting a "Twenty-first Century Biomedical Initiative" designed to double NIH funding over a ten-year period. We went to see her to ask whether the administration could make it a faster, five-year project. She said, "Go talk to people in the White House," and gave us a list.

We expended enormous amounts of energy just securing meetings, but we succeeded. One was with Vice President Al Gore, who opened the session by declaring, "I'll tell you right now, I'm for doubling NIH. Now, will you support a tax on tobacco to pay for it?" The tobacco tax was a sure loser in Congress, so we didn't sign on. Indeed, the tobacco tax did die. Clinton did call for a "biomedical initiative." He declared that "the twentieth century is the century of physics, but the twenty-first century will be the century of biology." But he still asked for NIH funding to be doubled over ten years, not five, and dropped even that goal after one year.

NIH2 dissolved after one last fiasco—a press conference in March 1999 to protest Clinton's latest lowball budget. There were no protocol foul-ups this time. Senator Specter came and was accorded his appropriate honored role. But after the event the *Washington Post's* media critic, Howard Kurtz, called to ask whether it was appropriate for me, as a journalist, to chair a lobbying organization. I said, "I believe in this cause, and if somebody doesn't like it, it's too bad." He quoted me in the paper. The next day the head of the Senate Periodical Gallery called and said that if I stayed on as NIH2 chairman I had to give up my press credentials. By the rules of the system, if I lost my congressional press pass, I'd lose my White House press pass and also my ability to cover national political conventions. So I resigned, and the group died.

But the cause succeeded. Specter, Mack, and Porter doggedly fought for and won congressional support for increases of more than 14 percent for NIH in fiscal years 1999 and 2000. I cheered them on in columns—publicizing, for instance, a report by the Joint Economic Committee, which Mack headed, on the dramatic savings already achieved by medical research. The polio vaccine, the report said, saves $30 billion every year in medical costs. Antibiotic treatments for tuberculosis save $5 billion, and a laser treatment for blindness caused by diabetes $1.5 billion. The death rate from AIDS had dropped by 60 percent, it said, and a $71 million NIH project on testicular cancer was curing 65 percent of those afflicted, saving $180 million every year.

In other columns I regularly urged increased funding for hospitals, especially teaching hospitals, which are going bankrupt because of miscalculated 1997 federal budget cuts. I opposed proposals put forward in Congress and by Vice President Gore that inevitably would lead to price controls on pharmaceuticals, which would inhibit investment and innovation by drug companies. It's true that drugs cost so much that some poor and elderly people can't afford them. However, the answer is not to have the government set prices, as Canada and Mexico do. No new drug discoveries come from there. One answer is to let those in need join insurance plans or other cooperatives that can bargain with pharmaceutical companies. Another is for the government to subsidize the effort. In columns, I argued that Republicans, including Bush, ought to be more generous in funding their prescription drug plans than they were.

On the other side of the 2000 presidential race, I wrote columns criticizing Bush for opposing federal funding of research using stem cells, the inner core of newly fertilized human embryos that can be converted into any other kind of cell. Stem cell research offers hope for curing a broad range of maladies, from spinal injuries to burns. Bush said he opposed the research because he is "pro-life," but I argued—as Bob Dole had done in 1992 in the fetal tissue fight—that using the cells to cure disease was the true pro-life position. Not only can stem cells cure the diseases of people who will otherwise die, including children, but the embryos to be used in federal research are those that have been left behind at in vitro fertilization clinics and are destined for destruction.

Besides writing columns, I kept nagging Bush's political and issues staff to get the candidate to make a major speech proposing a doubling of funding for medical research. I worked on Bush harder than Gore because I figured (wrongly) that Bush was going to win the presidency easily and because I thought that Gore, with his scientific bent, would require less convincing if he got elected.

In September 2000, Bush did come out for doubling, and with a rousing statement: "As president, I will fund and lead a medical moonshot to reach far beyond what seems possible today and discover new cures for age-old afflictions. . . . Our government will promote medical advances with new resources and new resolve." Bush's campaign staff produced a position paper that was amazingly thorough and sophisticated about the hopes that medical research might fulfill reasonably soon, including gene therapies for cystic fibrosis, Huntington's disease, and some forms of deafness and new drugs that strangle the blood vessels that feed tumors. The language on Parkinson's was pure music: "The world's leading neuroscientists have declared that Parkinson's can be cured within ten years—and what's learned in the process can help cure Alzheimer's, Huntington's, and other neurodegenerative diseases." Bush promised to finish the job that Hatfield, Porter, Specter, and Harkin had started in fiscal 1998, doubling the NIH budget to $27.5 billion by fiscal 2003. He promised to increase spending over ten years by $67 billion.

This was a great development, but I still harbored some doubts about Bush. First, if he stuck to his promise to the right-to-life movement and stopped NIH funding of stem cell research, he would be turning off one of the most promising rocket engines in his promised "moonshot." Second, even though his September speech was eloquent, the message was never repeated in the campaign, indicating it was not a core part of his program. And finally, he didn't promise to redouble the research budget in the five years after 2003. The $67 billion he budgeted would not pay for redoubling over ten years. Chances are good that only continued activism by research advocates will ensure that the promises of science are realized.

This is especially the case for brain research. Along with outer space, the human brain is one of the most exciting and mysterious territories in the universe. This one organ is the seat of consciousness, intelligence, emotion, and creativity, as well as the locus of mental illness and numerous physical ailments. But how it works, and sometimes doesn't, is only beginning to be discovered. In 2000, Congress took a step toward integrating the work of several NIH institutes that study the brain by establishing the National Neuroscience Research Center, which, fittingly, will be named after John Porter. What Clinton did for the Human Genome Project, it is in Bush's power to do for neuroscience.

Unfortunately, Congress's progress toward doubling NIH funding is no guarantee that Parkinson's funding will rise fast enough to produce an early cure. The tide is rising for medical research, and the Parkinson's boat is rising with it, but too slowly— far too slowly to save Milly. In 1998 I joined the advisory council that oversees the National Institute of Neurological Diseases and Stroke. Early the next year the new director of NINDS, Dr. Gerald Fischbach, gave an overview of brain science to the council and made the statement that Parkinson's could be cured within ten years. He did not say the same about any other disease. He said that Parkinson's discoveries could lead the way in curing other neurodegenerative diseases. Bush's staff, in effect, later quoted what Fischbach had said.

The Parkinson's community naturally hoped that Fischbach's

opinion would lead to something like a moonshot or a Manhattan Project for Parkinson's. Unfortunately, this did not happen. Parkinson's funding has increased, but by exactly how much, it is difficult to know. When members of Congress ask NIH, it responds that more than $150 million a year is being spent—"directly and indirectly." But bureaucrats at NIH acknowledge that the number includes any project that can be remotely connected to Parkinson's. In 1999 Joan Samuelson asked several Parkinson's researchers to analyze NIH's grants and come up with an accurate figure. They calculated that only about $53 million was being spent directly on Parkinson's, or $53 per victim. That was double the 1994 estimate, but still far short of the money being spent in 1999 on AIDS research ($1,800 per victim) or cancer ($400). And it was still far short of the $100 authorized in the Udall bill.

Michael J. Fox's announcement in late 1998 that he has Parkinson's changed the landscape both politically and psychologically. The boyish and beloved star of movies and TV sitcoms put the disease on the cover of countless magazines, including *People* and *Newsweek*, and made it the subject of dozens of network TV segments. The public now understood that this "old people's disease" afflicted young people, too. Michael was thirty-seven when he revealed that he had Parkinson's. He had been diagnosed at age thirty.

The minute he made his revelation, Parkinson's groups descended upon him, asking him to be their spokesman—meaning, of course, their fund-raiser. One group, he bemusedly recounted later, pitched him to join, but in the event he decided not to, urged him not to sign on with any other Parkinson's organization. The chairman of another group turned him off by badgering him to appear at its annual dinner. Joan wrote to him several times, but at first got no reply. Fox got interested in PAN, though, after hearing Mike Claeys, PAN's policy coordinator, talk about advocacy, lobbying, and politics. "It was clear he loves politics," Claeys said. Claeys, thirty-three, had been a congressional aide but was mesmerized on meeting Joan and spent the next five years as her major lobbying agent on Capitol Hill.

In 1999 Senator Thad Cochran of Mississippi, a new ally, urged Senator Specter to hold a hearing on Parkinson's. Specter, always eager for stars to appear before his subcommittee, asked Joan to see whether Fox would do so. She asked. He agreed, and she invited me to go with her and Claeys to brief Mike at his apartment in New York. I was instantly impressed by his total lack of pretentiousness and his keen awareness of how effectively his celebrity could be used to advance the Parkinson's cause. "This is not about me," he said. "I just want to win." He struck me as by far the nicest famous person I had ever met.

He did not seem to be having any trouble with Parkinson's symptoms that day, but he told us that a few weeks earlier his medicine had gone "off" on the set of *Spin City*. He'd retreated to his dressing room and turned on the cable channel MSNBC, which was running a retrospective on his acting career. He told us, "I appreciated it, but I know that's not what I want my legacy to be. I want my legacy to be what I do to beat Parkinson's disease." He also said he had quietly checked out Parkinson's groups—sometimes by anonymously logging into chat rooms on the Internet—and was impressed by what PAN was doing.

Specter's hearing was held on September 28, 1999, in the huge marble room in the Hart Senate Office Building where Milly and I had testified in 1995. Mike and Joan were witnesses along with Fischbach, the Pennsylvania Parkinson's activist Jim Cordy, and the famed Parkinson's scientist Bill Langston. I got there early and chatted with Mike in a holding room. He looked stiff and fidgety. I assumed that his morning dose of Sinemet had yet to take effect. Later he told Diane Sawyer in an ABC-TV interview that he'd purposely not taken his medicine so that the world would get some idea of what Parkinson's does to people. Joan had left her prepared statement back at her hotel and spent the time scribbling notes. Milly was wheeled to a front-row seat in the hearing room, which was packed with spectators, many wearing PD buttons, and lined with TV cameras. I sat next to her when the testimony began.

Mike was showing the effects of not having taken medicine. He shifted in his chair and joked that he had trouble turning pages. But his testimony was eloquent. He described how he'd originally tried to hide his symptoms, then decided to "soldier on," as many patients do, without revealing to the world that he had the disease. But, he said, "the time for quietly soldiering on is through. The war against Parkinson's is a winnable war, and I have resolved to play a role in that victory." He said he was "shocked and frustrated" to learn how meager an amount of money was spent on Parkinson's research. He praised Specter for working to double NIH funding, but said, "I implore you to do more for people with Parkinson's. Take up Parkinson's as if your life depended on it. Increase funding for Parkinson's research by $75 million over the current levels over the coming year." That was the sum that a research panel organized by PAN and the Parkinson's activist Jeffrey Martin said could fruitfully be spent on various areas of research. Specter said he thought that $75 million was "doable."

Fox finished on a personal note that was carried on practically every television news show in the nation that night. With the help of medicine, he said, he could still function as a young man, husband, father, and actor. "But I don't kid myself. That will change." He was gradually becoming more physically and mentally exhausted, he said, and was experiencing more tremor and rigidity. "I can expect in my forties to face challenges most people won't expect until their seventies or eighties, if ever. But with your help, if we all do everything we can to eradicate this disease, in my fifties I'll be dancing at my children's weddings."

Even though Mike's testimony was the news event of the day, Joan's was equally moving. She recalled visits she'd made to Mo Udall's hospital room with his daughter Anne, who had mordantly said the first time, "I guess I'm taking you to see your future." In 1991, Joan told the senators, Udall "had entered a stage that I haven't yet, which is the departure from society. He was still able to sit up in a wheelchair, and I could understand a few words that he was able to say with great difficulty." As she spoke about Udall, I thought that she was describing Milly, and I clutched her hand. Then Joan nearly brought me to tears when she said, "Two years later she took me back to see him. He was lying in bed, unable to move, unable to speak. And that was the living death, which is the next stage, which is then followed by death itself. That is the fate I look forward to with great fear and desperation, that I need to have a rescue from as soon as I can." Joan and Milly were diagnosed with Parkinson's the same year, but they have very different cases. Joan can walk, though sometimes she drags her leg, and she is one of the most articulate people alive. Milly's case is much more like Mo Udall's. She is much closer to "the living death."

After the hearing Milly met Fox, and they established a mutual admiration society that endures. Mike always asks about Milly whenever I see him, and Milly wants to know the details about every conversation I have with Mike. Mike says Milly is his hero.

Milly says that while she often wishes she were dead, she stays alive partly not to disappoint Mike.

Following their testimony, Mike and Joan went around Capitol Hill for a series of sessions with Senate and House leaders that demonstrated how starstruck these governmental grandees can be. Senate Majority Leader Trent Lott beamingly told him that $75 million more for Parkinson's was something he thought he could support, and he joked with Fox that he ought to run for the Senate as a Republican, having once played a young Reaganite, Alex P. Keaton, on the TV show *Family Ties*. Mike told him he wasn't yet an American citizen. He passed over the fact that, when he did become one—as he did the following year—he would vote as a liberal Democrat.

On the House side, Fox had what proved to be a portentous meeting with the chairman of the appropriations committee, Representative Bill Young, though it seemed surreal at the time. Young's wife, Beverly, wearing jeans and a faded, tattered sweatshirt, ushered in a dozen or so relatives, personal friends, and their children for individual pictures with Mike and also ran the substantive meeting at which Mike and Joan made their pitch for more funding. Specter, Lott, and Young did not come through with $75 million or any extra money. But Young saw to it that the next appropriation bill did contain language ordering NIH to perform its own strategic study of Parkinson's science and come up with a budget estimate for meeting the goal. That turned out to be $1 billion extra over five years, starting with $75 million in the first year—just what Joan's and Jeff Martin's experts' study had proposed. In yet a third meeting that day Representative Jerry Lewis of California, chairman of the defense appropriations subcommittee, promised to restore $10 million that had been cut from former Representative McDade's Pentagon research program on neurotoxins.

Fox and Joan left the Capitol high-fiving each other. Fox was thrilled to be involved in politics. They began working toward an alliance, and I became involved as an adviser. At one meeting in December 1999 at the offices of Lottery Hill Entertainment, Mike's production company in New York, Mike said he wanted to create a private foundation to foster Parkinson's research. He said he thought he could raise millions of dollars from his friends in the New York financial community and the entertainment industry. He mentioned Jeffrey Katzenberg of DreamWorks and Martin Scorsese, whose wife has Parkinson's, as people who might help. There was excitement in the room. It always had been a dream of Joan's, too, to do more than just advocacy and lobbying, but also to finance cutting-edge research that NIH might not pay for, accustomed as it was to supporting mainly proven investigators.

Mike asked about PAN's financial condition. As Joan's chief fund-raiser, I said that PAN would fall about $100,000 short of its budget before the next Udall dinner could replenish the till. After the meeting Mike disappeared into his private office for fifteen minutes, then emerged and called Joan in. He told her he'd been on the phone with his accountant to see whether he had a spare $100,000 he could give her. He did, and he wrote PAN a check.

In January Mike announced that he was leaving *Spin City* to devote himself to conquering Parkinson's. This produced a huge new burst of publicity—and an invitation from Hillary Clinton to sit in her box when President Clinton delivered his State of the Union message on January 27. I was sitting in Chicago's O'Hare Airport en route from the Iowa presidential caucuses to the Sundance Film Festival in Utah, where my daughter Alex was screening a short film. My cell phone rang. It was Mike. He said he was inclined to turn down Hillary's invitation. It would look like an endorsement of her senatorial candidacy, he said. I was a little startled, but in an instant I realized that he had shrewd judgment. I said, "You are absolutely right. All you'll get out of it is five minutes of face time with Hillary, if that. She'll promise you something for Parkinson's, but she'll lie just like Clinton did to Christopher Reeve. You'll just get used." Without accepting my invidious analysis, he skipped the State of the Union.

The next month I flew out to Los Angeles aboard the Disney Corporation's luxurious executive jet with Mike and his canny, generous partner at Lottery Hill, Danelle Black, to meet with Mike's lawyers and professional advisers about merging PAN into the Fox Foundation. On the way I told him all about Milly and her experience with Parkinson's, and we shared our experiences as recovering alcoholics. He told the group in Los Angeles, "We've made a lot of money together, and we've done great work. This is what I want to do now, and I want you to help me."

Mike's last *Spin City* episode was scheduled to run on May 24. We scheduled the Udall dinner for May 23 and decided to honor John Porter and Connie Mack. Mike said he would attend and would ask *Spin City* cast members and other friends to come, too, and swell the take. May 23 also became the date we'd announce the merger of PAN into the Michael J. Fox Foundation for Parkinson's Research.

For me, the spring of 2000 went by in a blaze. I was writing columns and doing Fox News commentaries on presidential politics, constantly making fund-raising and planning calls for the Udall dinner, and helping with strategy for the launch of the Fox Foundation, including a suggestion to *Newsweek* that it consider a cover story on Mike and Parkinson's. Mike's publicist, Nanci

Ryder, made the actual arrangements with *Newsweek* for exclusivity in return for the cover, which ran on May 22. And much more than me, Mike and his staff, and Joan and PAN's staff, put themselves on a forced march to find people who created the logo, web site, legal framework, public service ads, and phone banks in time for the launch.

The Udall dinner was transformed that year by Mike's presence. His dazzling *Spin City* co-star, Heather Locklear, was there along with cast members Richard Kind, Alan Ruck, and Connie Britton. The TV sports and entertainment broadcaster Pat O'Brien, who'd lost his mother to Parkinson's, served as emcee for the dinner. The Washington Hilton Hotel, often the site of Udall dinners, resembled a movie premiere that night, with reporters, TV crews, and spectators straining at rope lines to glimpse, photograph, and interview the stars. We sold more tickets and tables than we ever had before and filled the biggest hotel ballroom in D.C. Before turning the microphone over to Pat O'Brien, I joked that we had invented a new art form for Washington—the marriage-as-fund-raiser, with the guests paying to attend the wedding ceremony.

Romance and marriage analogies were the order of the evening. Introducing Mike, Joan said, "You know, your life can be going along pretty well, and all of a sudden this special someone comes along one day and knocks your socks off." The special day for her, she said, was September 28, when she and Fox visited Capitol Hill. "It was amazing and magic, and things are never going to be the same, thank goodness. So there's going to be a union, and as with the best of such situations, everything we have been doing will continue, only it will get better." She said that henceforth the Parkinson's effort would be "powered by the love

that this country has for this man—powered like no rocket anyone has ever seen." On a screen where Joan had been showing
slides of "PAN family" traditions and successes—including shots
of Milly testifying—she began showing pictures of Mike, and her
show ended with the PAN logo replaced by the new one of the
Fox Foundation.

When he took the stage Mike showed more effects of Parkinson's than most other people or I had ever seen before. His shoulders and hips swayed involuntarily, and he fumbled with his
papers. It made the moment all the more touching and dramatic:
Fox was among friends, supporters, and fellow victims. He didn't
have to hide. And he didn't. But he was, as always, funny, self-
deprecatory, and inspiring. He joked that "Joan and I share a common affliction . . . a hopeless addiction to lame metaphors," and
described a "whirlwind romance" that he said he hoped would be
followed by a "ten-year honeymoon, followed by an amicable dis-
solution celebrated by a huge party" when Parkinson's had a cure.
He kidded that he had wanted to name his foundation, not after
himself, but "PD Cure." He said his wife, the actress Tracy Pollan,
had torpedoed that idea with a one-word question: "Pedicure?"
But seriously, he said, "in light of the incredible dedication, commitment, and accomplishment of the Parkinson's Action Network, I am humbled to have my name attached to what you are
doing. And I promise to dedicate myself to living up to the honor
of serving this community."

Sadly, the union of PAN and the Michael J. Fox Foundation
did not last. Joan Samuelson, while an inspiring speaker and hard-
driving advocate, is not an administrator. Joan and the PAN staff
worked tirelessly, but after the dinner and over the summer of
2000, when the foundation should have gotten up and running,

raising and dispensing money, it was not doing so. Mike became impatient. Joan became defensive. The relationship frayed. I was busy watching the presidential campaign and working on this book and didn't understand what was happening until it was too late. I listened to both sides but could not reconcile them. In the late fall PAN and the Fox Foundation formed separate, cooperative entities—Joan and PAN to continue with advocacy and lobbying, the Fox Foundation to raise and distribute money for research. I'm honored to be on the board of both organizations, but sad that they are not one.

In the fall, just before the 2000 election, Mike wrote an op-ed column in the *New York Times* pointing out the differences between George Bush and Vice President Al Gore on the issue of embryonic stem cell research—Bush remained against it, Gore was for it—and urging that the research be allowed to continue in order to save lives. Because Joan, Mike Claeys, and I supplied background data for the piece, I was encouraged to think that cooperation between PAN and Mike would continue. And indeed it did when Bush became president, as we strategized on what to do after Bush hinted that he might issue an executive order banning federal money for stem cell research. Bush heard from numerous disease advocates—including Connie Mack—urging him not to stop the research. And he did not, at least immediatley, ordering a study of the issue instead. Mike decided he would try to see Bush along with Joan, urge him to allow stem cell research to proceed, and call upon him to launch a neurological "moonshot" to discover the secrets of the brain. Mike wants to tell him that he could be the president who presides over the conquest of Parkinson's.

This disease will be conquered. The crucial breakthrough may come as the result of a grant from the Michael J. Fox Foundation. Or it may come as the result of an NIH or Defense Department grant made possible by PAN's lobbying. Conceivably it could come as the result of work by researchers on a wholly different disease who got their support because the overall federal research budget was doubled. All those who work for an end to Parkinson's and other terrible diseases are God's workers. I am proud to be one of them. And I hope that President Bush will join us.

8

Losing Milly

The bride, Nicole Reyes, and the groom, Michael Dadich, and their attendants seemed blissfully unaware that a parallel festivity was taking place at their wedding reception outside of Chicago in September 2000. It was a reunion of the Roulettes and the Latin Dons. The honored guest—bathed in affection, laughingly recalled memories, and blinked-back tears—was Milly. Her old neighborhood girlfriends and guyfriends are all middle-class suburbanites now, filled out and gray. They see each other from time to time at weddings and funerals, but when the word got around that Milly was coming to the wedding of Mona Reyes's daughter, calls poured in from the whole gang asking for invitations.

I have not seen Milly so happy in years. I pushed her in her wheelchair from table to table, with her foster sister Lori videotaping as I asked her old pals for their favorite Milly memories. There was a constant theme: as president of the Roulettes, she was bossy, "the dictator," "the headmistress," but with everyone's welfare and respectability in mind. She established rules: no smoking in public, no kissing boys in public, no French kissing ever, no drinking, no swearing. Don't ditch classes, get your homework done before you go out, and graduate and go to college. Violators—there were lots of violators, they mirthfully reported—had to pay a fine of twenty-five cents per offense, which was used to build up the Roulette treasury so the girls could buy club jackets. Milly also organized hayrides and dances in church basements to raise money.

Ex-Dons reported that she'd also tried to boss them around but was even less successful. Besides drinking, some of their activities—petty theft, stealing a car, robbing drunks—could have had consequences, and no one dared tell Milly about them then, and they even hesitated to tell her about them now. To put her down in the old days, one of the guys used to pinch her nose, knowing that she thought it was too big and that she hated it when he did that. He ceremonially did it at the party, causing everyone to roar, especially Milly. It developed that Milly once had a crush on one of the guys, green-eyed Rudy Ortega, who'd invited himself to the wedding from California to see her. "She always wanted him to kiss her," Lori said, "but he never would." He finally did that night, and Milly looked like a schoolgirl.

It's fair to say there might have been no wedding that day without Milly. The bride's father, Danny Reyes, said his favorite Milly story was that when he returned to Chicago from serving in the army, his old girlfriend, Mona, didn't want to see him or even talk to him. At a beach party Milly told Mona: "Go kiss him." She did, they got back together, and they've been married for forty years. And this was not the only match made by Milly, her friends said. In recognition of the leadership and judgment she'd shown in her youth, and the courage she was obviously showing now—unable to speak, only to laugh, receive hugs, and be there—these old friends swathed her in love and made her bloom. To see it made me as happy, too, as I have been in years.

Then, on her first day back in Washington, Milly went to see a dentist about her latest project—orthodontics. Her lower front teeth have always been mildly crooked—West Side Chicago kids didn't get braces—but Parkinson's has caused her chin to recede and her teeth have become more misaligned. She has somehow convinced herself that if her teeth are straightened, the effects of Parkinson's will be less visible. This almost surely won't work, but I can refuse Milly nothing, so she is getting braces at age sixty-one. Vanity is a sign that, in her tormented inner debate about whether to keep fighting or give up, the balance still favors life.

I take joy in such signs because I desperately do not want to lose her. I am happy that Milly pores through the catalogs that come in the mail and each season orders clothing to keep herself smartly dressed. She cannot be heard on the phone, so she shows Grelanda or Felly what she wants and hands them a credit card. She takes excursions to Saks and one day racked up purchases worth $8,000; that time I did refuse and made her take it all back, or almost all. Afterward she justified the spree to her friend Netty Graulich on the grounds that, "as the wife of Morton Kondracke, I deserve to be well dressed." She is forever showing grit. When the Siegels bought an elegant brownstone in our neighborhood, Milly insisted on fully inspecting it—every room and closet on all four floors and the roof deck, with me helping her mount and descend the stairs. When she's wheeled through a doorway, she insists on reaching around to turn out the light and shut the door, even though she's liable to hurt her arm in the process. She wants her eyebrows tweezed. She's never satisfied with the way I brush her hair and invariably redoes it herself. When there was a reception for Michael J. Fox at the 2000 Republican convention in Philadelphia, she insisted on being driven up from Washington to attend and had her picture taken, beaming, with Muhammad Ali. Even though drugs and operations have failed to arrest her Parkinson's, she is willing to try anything that might work.

As Milly is regularly brave, I fleetingly indulge in fantasies that she might recover. One day when I was giving her a shower I noticed that her hair is not all white; in the back there are some strands of black. I thought, *Could this be the first hint of a reversal of the Parkinson's?* It was no such thing, of course, and I knew it. But there are other moments. Once in a while she will speak absolutely clearly. The Old Milly will be back for an instant, telling me to phone the girls, saying she wants to make this or that trip or reminding me to send flowers to somebody. She can never walk unaided, but sometimes she moves smoothly, especially on stairs. Ordinarily she needs to have her food chopped up or pureed and she can't manipulate a fork or spoon by herself and has to be fed. But sometimes she'll insist on having mussels or barbecued ribs for dinner and gets them down without choking. Other times, she pushes away help and manipulates her own fork. Whenever any such thing happens, I think, *Could the disease be turning around somehow?*

Alas, it is not. The flashes of hope disappear and the reality dominates: my wife is slipping away from me. She is dying, slowly but inexorably. It's progressively harder for her to eat solid foods, and if she tries to drink from a glass it usually goes down the wrong pipe, making her gag. Often she has trouble even drawing liquids up through a straw. For unexplained reasons, she drools some of the time, but other times not. She is able to make herself understood only intermittently. Her voice has no volume, and she has difficulty forming intelligible words. She remains willing to try any experimental procedure that might improve her condition, but the doctors are running out of ideas.

It grieves me to look at what is happening to her, but often my heart is filled with awe that she is so beautiful—radiant, almost luminous. Her white hair, cut short, makes her look like an angel. Her skin is smooth. Sometimes her jaw relaxes and she sits with her brow furrowed and her eyes closed tight, making her look like an aged philosopher deep in meditation. Other times, eyes closed peacefully, she looks like a child asleep or a saint in a mystical reverie, almost transfigured. But my favorite expression is Milly wide-eyed, sharing a joke. I get that look when I tease her about being an indiscriminate Democrat, when I remind her of one of the many times over the years when I was wrong and she was right, or if I suggest that perhaps tonight would be a good night for Viagra.

Her taste is impeccable. The dresses she buys tend to be loose-fitting, and her trousers usually have elastic tops to make it easy to take her to the bathroom. But they are stylish. She likes fine jewelry, and I like to promise her that I will buy things for her—a ring for Christmas, a necklace for her birthday, diamond earrings for our wedding anniversary. One of our favorite things to do together is to go buy them. One of my favorite things to do is to buy them without her and surprise her.

One day a local TV channel doing a piece on Michael J. Fox showed an old clip of an interview with Milly when her hair was dyed. She told me she wanted it dark again and had Felly make an appointment. I had to argue and enlist her friends, Grelanda, Alex, and Andréa to convince her she looked much better all-white. Milly also likes to go on trips—to Chicago, to the annual

Parkinson's Unity Walk in New York, to Mexico, on ocean cruises. And I plan them. Purchases, trips, and visits from our daughters are the current version of the Old Milly's projects. In fact, they are more important. Anticipation and fulfillment help keep her alive.

Milly can still make me angry. Sometimes I'm exhausted from work and she decides at 11:00 P.M. that she wants to rearrange her clothes closet. I yell at her that for God's sake why couldn't she do this during the day with one of her ladies? But I end up doing what she wants just to make her happy. I do not know how much longer I will have her, so I treasure tasks I used to find unpleasant. If she needs to go to the bathroom, we "dance" to the toilet, and it's a chance for me to hold her. When I change her disposable underwear, I view it as a chance to do stretching exercises. We make a joke out of the enemas she needs three or four times a week. I tell her, "I know you'd do the same for me," and I get the wide-eyed look that I love. Milly usually wakes up earlier than I do and immediately wants to turn the TV on. If she can't find the remote, I hunt for it, click it, and bury my head under a pillow. I tell her to report to me if something's happened I should know about.

Because of communications difficulties, I do not know completely what she is thinking. We tried microphones and voice amplifiers, but they didn't work because Milly can't articulate well. We've tried two rounds of Silverman Method speech therapy, which involves deep-breathing exercises, but they've produced no long-term improvement. Singing sometimes warms up Milly's voice for a few words of speech, but the next ones can't be understood. We have tried various computer-based voice synthesizers, but they are either too complicated or require too much manual dexterity for Milly to operate. Stephen Hawking, the British astrophysicist stricken with ALS, uses one of these machines. But when Milly and I tried something like it, we concluded that one had to have Hawking's IQ to program it. Also, the electronic voices built into these machines are hard to understand at best, and given Milly's tendency not to use a space bar between words, what came out was gibberish.

I thought at one stage, what about magnetized letters, the kind parents put up on the refrigerator door to help children learn the alphabet? I got some at a toy store but couldn't find a metal board for Milly to arrange them on. On a visit, her sister Alex suggested a cookie sheet. A good idea, but it proved unwieldy. I bought several Scrabble sets, but it was hard for Milly to move letters very fast. I bought a children's computer, but when Milly touched any letter it raced repetitiously across the screen.

Finally a speech therapist suggested a paper alphabet chart, laminated in plastic, and we've been using it ever since, though it's sometimes hard to follow as Milly drags her finger across the page. Sometimes, too, she spells words backward or scrambles them. She means "WHAT" but spells "HATW." Recently I've rigged up laptops with desktop keyboards in the kitchen and bed-room, and she communicates by punching out words in forty-eight-point type, though she often hits the wrong key and never uses the space bar. And we've recently acquired a nifty small com-puter, an AlphaSmart, which we take with us outside the house, though it presents the same problems. Milly cannot nod or shake her head well, so she raises one finger if the answer to a question is yes and two if it's no. We play Twenty Questions a lot. I cannot hear her at all if we are driving, so we've invented a system: she holds my index finger, and I run through the alphabet. She squeezes when I get to the right letter. It takes a while to spell out a message, but the system works.

The thoughts she expresses now are perhaps a quarter as complex as those of the Old Milly. She mainly tells me what she wants—to go to the bathroom or kitchen or to the movies or a bookstore. Or to get her candy or give her money. She tells me to call the girls, and when I do she listens in on an extension and taps out messages for me to relay. Mainly, she writes, "WHENAREYOUCOMINGHOME?" She has me call up friends who have been sick. She tells me which political candidates she likes, and we bet each other $1,000 on election outcomes—it's the same bank account, after all—but she doesn't carry on extended political arguments any longer. Nor does she make her old penetrating character evaluations of other people.

Once I feared that Milly, like many Parkinson's victims, was descending into dementia. One neurologist looked at an MRI and said he believed she had Lewy body disease, a condition in which free radicals attack the cerebral cortex and lower IQ. When she had her second operation at Emory, though, Dr. DeLong looked at his extensive MRI collection and said that he saw evidence only of damage in the cerebellum, which controls balance. Andréa, then a second-year medical student, agreed with him.

To get a later reading on all this and help determine whether any other invasive treatments made sense—a fetal transplant, for instance—we went to New York University's North Shore Hospital on Long Island for a PET scan in the summer of 2000. This procedure, using radioactive isotopes injected into the blood, yields pictures showing the level of metabolic activity in various parts of the brain. In the picture, active parts turn up red. Damaged, inactive parts come up blue-violet. Milly's PET scan showed violet areas in the basal ganglia and striatum, where movement signals are transmitted, which is usual in Parkinson's victims. But it also showed a disconcerting amount of loss in the cerebellum and the cortex. It was as though acid had eaten away at parts of her brain. The several doctors who looked at the pictures have confirmed once again that Milly has no ordinary case of Parkinson's.

Exactly what it is and what's caused it, none of them seems to know. At NIH, Dr. Chase looked at the pictures and said, "If I had to put a name on it, I'd call it cortical basal ganglionic degeneration. I can give you a paper on the subject, but you'll see, it doesn't say anything about causes or consequences because we don't know anything. The truth is, we don't know what Milly has, and if we did know we wouldn't know what to do about it." Another NIH researcher, Dr. David Goldstein, said that he thinks Milly has Shy-Drager syndrome, also known as multi-system atrophy. Like Chase, he said that no one understands this condition either. The PET scan did seem to establish that the currently available Parkinson's treatments—and those on the immediate horizon—will do her very little good. Fetal and stem cell transplants, new surgical techniques, and most new pharmaceuticals are all designed to deal with classic Parkinson's, the absence of dopamine. They will control freezing and tremor. Some may correct for loss of balance. But the combination of these symptoms, plus loss of speech and swallowing ability and cortical damage—"Milly Syndrome," as Mahlon DeLong called it—is beyond current science.

This means that, absent a miracle, Milly will continue to deteriorate. In early 2001, it appeared that a small miracle might be under way. But it could prove to be a great disappointment instead. In late 2000, Dr. Goldstein casually told Dr. Chase that there was anecdotal evidence that yohimbine, a drug derived from an African evergreen tree that's used to treat male impotence, helped strengthen the speech of people with Shy-Drager syndrome. In February of 2001, the two of them conspired to fit Milly into a study that Goldstein was doing on heart responses to yohimbine, which increases the body's production of norepineph-rine, a substance akin to adrenaline. They gave her a PET scan of the heart to satisfy that protocol and infused a very small dose of yohimbine intravenously. Within seconds, Milly's speech became intelligible—still weak, still slurred, but understandable.

When I got home, I was amazed and overjoyed, as were Alex and Andréa, who both happened to be in town at the time. The level of our discourse wasn't profound, but when Milly told us what had happened that day, we could understand her from a few feet away. The next day, however, the effect began to wear off, and I had to put my ear close to her face to make out what she was saying. Within two days she again could not be understood.

The obvious next step was to increase the dosage and see what would happen, but this did not fit into Dr. Goldstein's proto-col. So Dr. Chase designed a new study to see what oral dose of yohimbine might restore her speech and whether there were any side effects. So far, however, oral yohimbine has failed to produce any positive results. The intravenous experiment initially gave us great hope that Milly would be able to take yohimbine pills every day and speak. The experiments are still under way. If they suc-ceed they could transform the way Milly lives. She could gossip, make phone calls, and tell people what she thinks. She would no longer be isolated. And her swallowing might improve. The prospect thrills me. On the other hand, if the experiment fails it would be a cruel letdown—a great hope dashed.

Even at the best, however, yohimbine can not cure Parkinson's disease. Looking further for experimental treatments—miracles—Dr. Chase has found suggestions in some literature that a com-mon antibiotic, minocycline, may arrest apotosis, the process by which cells kill themselves in Parkinson's and kindred diseases. Conceivably, this drug could slow the progression of her illness, though it has yet to be tried in humans. There is no downside to trying this, Chase says, so when the yohimbine experiment is finished, he will try minocycline. And Milly, of course, is game for it. She is game for anything.

If that does not work, Chase says, hope may lie with so-called neurotophic factors, proteins that seem to repair neurological damage when injected into the brains of animals. So far, however, these substances haven't worked in humans. Moreover, the procedure for administering them—through a tube into the brain—is dangerous enough that it's been tried only on patients with dread conditions such as progressive supranuclear palsy (PSP), which kills its victims in five years or less. I have no doubt that if Milly were convinced that this procedure was her only hope for life, she would try it, too.

The existence of mysterious complications like Parkinson's-plus, Shy-Drager syndrome, cortical basal ganglionic degeneration, and PSP is further reason for an all-out research effort centered on the brain. For Milly and me, though, Chase's reminders of the research progress currently being made—or promised— have only heightened the excruciating sense that we are in a race against time—and that we are losing.

After the Reyes-Dadich wedding in Chicago, one of Milly's childhood friends, Helen Metoyer, organized the Roulettes and the Dons into a prayer circle for her and sent out instructions for saying rosaries on her behalf. Milly was touched by the gesture. She had left the Catholic Church decades ago, but we found old rosary beads in a drawer and she began praying, though on much the same premise as she agreed to take yohimbine and will try minocycline: she'll try anything.

Helen's initiative made me wonder why I, supposedly so much more faithful than Milly, have so seldom prayed for a miracle. I pray fervently and often for deliverance from petty problems—

"Please, God, let me not have lost my car keys"—and also for the success of career ventures and for the safety of my children. I have prayed for help for myself in taking care of Milly. I have prayed that Milly could have peace of mind in coping with her condition. But since her diagnosis, I have rarely prayed for her rescue. I believe that prayers are often answered. I believe that I have seen them answered. Yet somehow a cure for Milly seemed to be beyond what I imagined God could or would deliver. Helen's gesture—and the full recognition that I was losing Milly—caused me to resolve that I would pray every day for her cure and for God to forgive me for not asking Him sooner. Yohimbine may be an answer to those prayers. At least, it would give human contact back to Milly. That would be an enormous blessing.

And yet I do not trust that a miracle will be forthcoming that will save her life and restore her fully. I can't. Milly and I both must deal with reality as we perceive it, and with our fears. Before we went up to Long Island for the PET scan of her brain, Milly expressed apprehension that it would show mental deterioration. She wrote on the computer, "I THINK IM LOSING MY INTELLIGENCE. MY WORLD IS GETTING NARROW." Reviewing the PET scan pictures, I asked various doctors out of Milly's earshot whether what they saw implied lost cognitive ability. The answer was, in effect, yes. "But how much or where this is going, we can't tell. What you see is what you have," one of them said.

I definitely see diminution. On the other hand, it's crushingly evident that much of the savvy, wise, and tough Old Milly still lives in her wasting body and inside her head. For example, we had dinner one evening with a very liberal friend who expressed regret that he couldn't watch me on TV because his cable system doesn't carry Fox News. Milly tapped out the message on her AlphaSmart: "THAT'S GOOD IF YOU SAW WHAT HE SAYS YOU WOULD HATE HIM." After we saw the movie *The Talented Mr. Ripley*, I said to her that I couldn't understand how Gwyneth Paltrow's character, a smart writer, could be in love with a cad, played by Jude Law. She slowly spelled the message out on her letterboard: "E-V-E-R-Y-O-N-E K-N-O-W-S T-H-A-T Y-O-U-N-G W-O-M-E-N O-F-T-E-N F-A-L-L F-O-R S-H-I-T-S." I said, "*You* did—me." She gave me her wide-eyed smile, but I added quickly, "But you made me not-a-shit. Everyone becomes a better person because of you."

Well, not everyone. Milly once had a huge cadre of Washington friends, people who came to her for free advice about husbands, children, and other relationships. Of these, many have remained close and loyal. Jill Schuker comes to visit Milly every week, calls often, and arranges birthday and anniversary parties. Jill says that she and Milly communicate almost telepathically, their friendship is so deep. Mark and Judy Siegel bring food, invite us to their beach house, and do Thanksgiving, Passover, and July Fourth. Netty Graulich, Milly's old sewing teacher, takes Milly to the theater and for long dinners. Milly pecks out advice for Netty, and Netty always allows Milly to unburden her most desperate fears. Terry Schaefer, who has moved to New York, writes often to tell Milly how much she loves her. Gloria Doyle invites her to lunch and to tea. Another friend, Susan Lee, takes yoga instruction with Milly, and they have lunch and shop together. Milly's former psychotherapy partner, Sue Bailey, is always up for a movie. Some others, including the old Tunlaw Road wives, stay in touch, call to ask how Milly is, and sometimes gather for a dinner. Other old friends e-mail good wishes or call on the phone, offering to stop by when I am at home. These people, I assume, are afraid to be alone with Milly because they don't know how to communicate or don't know what to say to her.

Some people, however, have abandoned her. I phone these former neighbors and professional colleagues to say Milly misses them. Jill and other close friends call and write to them. They promise to call or visit. But they don't. I can understand why. She cannot be understood on the phone. Carrying on a conversation with her in person takes patience and effort. Needy people can't get their needs met easily by Milly anymore. They have to give. I understand what's going on, but it's hard to forgive them because Milly feels so hurt that they've dropped her. Yohimbine offers the promise that these people will come back. I know that Milly will welcome them. It's the way she is.

Milly reads books, likes movies, and has favorite TV shows, including *Oprah*—whose recommended books she always buys— and *Who Wants to Be a Millionaire?* Each time the show is ending and Regis Philbin refers to the 800 number for prospective contestants, Milly points to the screen and whispers, "Call!" I tell her that if I ever got on I'd miss a $200 pop culture question and disappoint her horribly. This is another occasion when she gives me her wide-eyed, knowing laugh. She also always remembers where things are in the house, including objects I put away and then forget. She remembers everyone's birthday and other special occasions and insists on sending flowers. She loves it when she can prove her memory is sharper than mine.

Milly has much to complain about, but she rarely complains. She once said to me that "suffering doesn't make you a better person. It makes you worse. You think about yourself all the time." This may apply to her, but it has less effect than it would for others. Unlike some people who suffer, she does not inflict her suffering on others—especially me. She tells me on her letterboard that she's angry if I leave her alone too long at a party or if I leave her on a Saturday or Sunday in the care of someone who doesn't drive. She lets me know if she thinks a caregiver is ignoring her. These are all legitimate issues to raise, though. She does not abuse anyone.

But she is deeply unhappy. Milly sometimes tells me—and others more than me—that she wants to commit suicide or die soon. One day she wrote to me on her letterboard: "I C-A-N-T T-A-L-K O-R W-A-L-K I D-O-N-T W-A-N-T T-O L-I-V-E L-I-K-E T-H-I-S." Another time she wrote: "N-E-V-E-R T-O E-A-T A H-O-T D-O-G A H-A-M-B-U-R-G-E-R O-R A S-A-L-A-D O-R B-E A-B-L-E T-O T-A-L-K I-S I-N-T-O-L-E-R-A-B-L-E." In a restaurant she painstakingly wrote out on the AlphaSmart, "I have been thinking about dying. You make me very happy, but I wonder how much longer God is going to make me suffer."

Incidents constantly occur that magnify her misery. We were at a noisy book-signing party for a good friend, and when people came up to talk to Milly, they could not make out what she was saying. So they quickly moved on. We'd brought her Alpha-Smart, but its battery was low and it conked out. I scribbled out a makeshift alphabet chart on a piece of paper and knelt by her chair to interpret for her, but few people had the patience to stay for long as she slowly traced out letters. As a result, Milly spent the evening essentially isolated and alone. When we got home, she told me, "I couldn't talk to anyone. I don't want to live anymore."

A worse incident occurred at NIH. For a moment, Felly left Milly sitting at a cafeteria table in her wheelchair. Her eyes evidently were closed. An enormous woman at the next table said something to Milly. When Milly didn't respond, because she couldn't, the woman screamed out that Milly was unconscious.

The woman yelled for help, pulled Milly out of her chair, and laid her out on the floor. Milly wanted to protest, but couldn't. An emergency crew rushed in. Felly ran up and said that Milly was fine, but couldn't speak because of Parkinson's disease. The crew paid her no mind. They checked Milly's vital signs, which were normal, but nonetheless hoisted her onto a stretcher and rushed her to an emergency room. She was quickly released, but she was shaken. "I felt like I was locked in a cage," she told me that night. "I couldn't do anything." She started to cry. I hugged her, but she broke into sobs. "I want to die," she said.

For Milly, even contemplating the future is bleak. As we were concluding our annual August week in Wisconsin with Lori and Jerry Long in 2000, I suggested we might go on a Christmas–New Year's ocean cruise with them in 2001. Afterward in our bedroom, Milly began weeping. "I want to die soon," she said on her Alpha-Smart. "I do not intend to be alive in 2002."

I used to be speechless at such moments. Or I would say, "You can't die. It would devastate the girls." Or, "You've got to see Andréa through medical school." The truth is that there are fleeting moments when I wish that Milly would die. I fantasize about a new life, post-Milly, post-Parkinson's, maybe with another woman who I can walk around Paris with, talk to in a normal way, and share retirement with. I confess that I sometimes indulge the fantasy to the extent of wondering about life with this or that particular woman I know. I also fantasize, though, that when Milly dies I'll contract melanoma or have a heart attack and follow her soon after, God having no more missions for me. In yet another idle daydream I marry a woman who shortly comes down with Parkinson's or an even worse chronic disease, like Alzheimer's or aggressive cancer. This is the future I would least want and one that would sorely test my faith. Yet I realize that if I did marry again in my mid- or late sixties, death is a challenge I would have to face again—hers or mine.

I never get very far with any of these scenarios because, as a stoic, I know that I can't possibly predict what my fate will be. I'm sure that what does happen will be completely different from anything I've fantasized or dreaded. As a faithful stoic, I leave the future in God's hands because I must. "The Author" will write the play. I merely hope that I can handle the part, whatever it is, with His help.

I have never discussed any of these fantasies with Milly. Typically, though, she has tried to engineer my future. "WHEN I DIE," she once tapped out on a laptop, "I WANT YOU TO STAY IN THE APARTMENT. IT WILL GIVE THE GIRLS A HOME." The truth is that Alex and Andréa don't regard our D.C. condominium as home at all. Like Milly, they still miss our house in Chevy Chase. More embarrassingly, twice Milly has said to different unmarried women friends in my presence, "When I die, I want you to marry Morton." In both cases, in unison, we've said, "Milly, shut up!"

Some friends have suggested that I should perhaps "develop a relationship" with another woman. Sometimes they genuinely just mean "talk, have lunch." Other times they are suggesting that I have an affair. One well-intentioned person recounted to me the story of a friend of hers who thought of leaving his wife but decided to stick with her when she was diagnosed with cancer. He fell in love with another woman and carried on a discreet affair with her for years, finally marrying her when his wife died. I quickly told this friend that my situation wasn't remotely analogous because I had never considered leaving Milly before she got sick and I've never been tempted to get involved with anyone else. Nor has anyone shown the slightest interest in me.

I won't deny that I feel lonely for intimate conversation, for someone to discuss my worries with and be nurtured by. My wonderful therapist, Dorree Lynn, has helped me get my narcissism under control, accept advice and praise, overcome the chronic mild depression that had me on Prozac for several years, kick away my preoccupations with status, and realize that my feelings of sadness over Milly's condition are entirely appropriate. Of course, two sessions a week don't substitute for long talks and long walks. I do tell Milly when I get home every night what I have done and what I'm worried about—some days it's the money in our checking account, and other days it's my boredom with politics and my vain wish to do something else professionally, like write novels or biographies. She listens, but I do not get a lot back—certainly not the challenging and penetrating advice Milly gave me when she was well. And until recently we talked hardly at all about what obviously tortured us both: Milly's deterioration and where it was heading.

In 1999 Dorree—who's also Milly's therapist—told me that Milly felt I was refusing to face up to the prospect of her dying. Dorree said that I was being selfish—forcing Milly to face death alone. She was absolutely right. In reality, I thought about the subject constantly but was afraid to talk to Milly for fear she would think I wanted her to die. I also was avoiding the pain that her thoughts about death would cause me. And I was petrified by what I thought were the only two options available. One was (and is) that we would do nothing and Milly would become like Mo Udall, spending years nourished through a feeding tube and, perhaps, eventually be warehoused in a nursing home. The only other option, I thought, was to use one of the techniques described in the book *Final Exit* to effect her suicide.

Milly and I started talking about her death in joint sessions with Dorree, and the first of these only increased my terror. Using her letterboard, Milly talked only about suicide. "I T-H-I-N-K A-B-O-U-T D-Y-I-N-G E-V-E-R-Y D-A-Y," she said. "F-O-R M-Y-S-E-L-F I W-O-U-L-D D-O I-T S-O-O-N B-U-T I D-O-N-T W-A-N-T T-O D-I-S-A-P-P-O-I-N-T O-T-H-E-R-S L-I-K-E M-I-C-H-A-E-L J F-O-X H-E T-H-I-N-K-S I-M A H-E-R-O-I-N-E."

With Dorree present, Milly poured out her feelings in a way that she rarely did when we were alone. On either the computer or the letterboard, she said in different sessions, "I do nothing every day. I can't talk in Bible study or movie group. I can't walk, and I can't eat. I don't know how you can love a mannequin." One day she said, "I'd like to get a fetal transplant and die on the operating table." Another time she wrote, chillingly, "Your love is not enough. I want to kill myself. I'm afraid, but I'm more afraid that I won't be able to move to do it." I asked her whether she wanted me to collect information and materials. She said, "Yes."

For months I lay awake nights and early mornings playing out strategies for the *Final Exit* option, becoming more panicky each time I did so. I dwelled on the rumor that Jacqueline Kennedy Onassis, stricken with terminal cancer, allegedly ended her own life with her loved ones gathered around her. But she was connected (I figured) with Fifth Avenue doctors who would have quietly prescribed the right medicine and signed her death certificate so that no questions were asked. Where would *I* find Seconal or Nembutal? I couldn't imagine any doctor I knew helping me.

When we lived in Chevy Chase, a kid down the street killed himself with a combination of over-the-counter medicines washed down with white wine. How could I find out what he'd used? Ask his parents? Look at his board of health records? Some friends suggested that I look for suicide information on the Internet, but not use my own computer, lest a record remain on the hard drive.

When I actually bought the book *Final Exit* I found it of little help: get a stash of barbiturates, it says, and mix them with pudding. Or take lots of Valium and put a plastic bag over your head.

After telling Milly I would get information and materials, I spent months in a state of near-terror trying to figure out what to do. If it were me, I thought, *I'd do the Valium–plastic bag thing.* But Milly couldn't do that without my help. If she opted for that— and insisted on it—would I really assist her? Could I stay in the apartment and watch her gasp, thrash, turn purple, and die? What would I tell the police afterward? Could I lie and tell them I'd gone out for a jog and found her dead when I got back? Could I pull that off? Would I go to jail? Maybe, I thought, I should just buy a gun somewhere and make it a mercy killing–suicide. I even thought about places in our apartment where I could do this and create the least possible cleanup problem.

At the end of most of these fevered scenario-plottings, I fervently prayed for help. I asked God, "Does this mission of Yours, 'taking care of Milly,' necessitate my killing her and maybe standing trial, ending my own future?" I decided, with a touch of shame but with conviction, that if killing Milly was what the mission demanded, I would not fulfill it. I would not go to jail. And of course, I would not commit a murder-suicide.

I believe that God speaks and acts through others—angels, as it were—and I believe I received a merciful gift through Milly's and my wise friend, Sue Bailey, a doctor who formerly was the assistant secretary of defense for health and head of the National Highway Transportation Safety Board. She said that, if Milly really wanted to end her own life, the way to do it would be to wait until a feeding tube became necessary. Milly could refuse it, enter a hospice, receive morphine to relieve discomfort, and starve to death. Afterward Milly and I talked about what Sue had said, and Milly said that this seemed the best alternative to her. We contacted our lawyer and had Milly's living will adjusted to permit her (or me as her agent) specifically to refuse a feeding tube as well as other artificial life-sustaining procedures. I also visited a hospice, the Washington Home, and arranged to get help if this is what Milly is determined to do when the time comes.

I was reassured by a doctor, a counselor at the hospice, and literature I read that death by starvation is not painful if the patient doesn't take liquids except to keep the mouth moistened. Food deprivation causes proteins and fat to burn up, inducing a process called ketosis, which produces euphoria and dampens discomfort. Giving the patient liquids causes swelling and pain; dehydration results in a clouding of consciousness. Death occurs in about six weeks through starvation alone, or in about three weeks through a combination of starvation and dehydration.

The hospice option came as a gift, a blessing, greatly easing my mind about how Milly might die. It delivered me from having to contemplate the horrific *Final Exit* suicide options. In fact, I think the growth of the hospice movement in America largely obviates the suicide issue—and the assisted-suicide issue—for the terminally ill, except for those in unbearable pain. If people can starve themselves to death peacefully, why would they (or their doctors) have to administer barbiturates to do it? As hospice literature argues, refusing or withholding food and water allows a natural death to happen.

Even so, what lies ahead is agony. Milly and I got a glimpse of it in Bill Moyers's PBS series on death and dying. In one episode a veterinarian with ALS contemplated using animal medicines in his possession to kill himself but let the opportunity slip because he waited until he could no longer swallow. His wife would not administer poison, and he finally realized that he was going to choke to death or die by starvation. Milly turned to me and whispered, "Is this what is going to happen to me?" The question, the closest we have yet come to speaking of the reality of her dying, struck me like an electric shock. I said, inadequately, "Yes, I think, something like that, but it will be a longer time coming. ALS is much faster than Parkinson's."

Of course, there is no way of telling how much time we have until we face the feeding tube decision—which I cannot bring myself to think of as the "starvation" decision. I hope that the time is measured in years, not months. I judge that I would have some warning if Milly started to need frequent Heimlich maneuvers to stop her from choking on food caught in her windpipe.

I have had to perform the maneuver three times in the past eighteen months. These are occasions of momentary terror, and I remember each one vividly. Milly had been urging me for years to arrange to be a speaker on an ocean cruise, and finally I was invited to do so during the Christmas–New Year's holidays in 1999–2000. It was a delightful time for us—traveling for three weeks from Florida, through the Panama Canal, and up the Pacific Coast to Los Angeles. Milly and I spent virtually every moment together. Alex and Andréa joined us for part of the cruise and gave me short breaks to work on my speeches or exercise. At lunch on a fantail deck of the ship one day off Mexico, Milly insisted on having a cracker-and-cheese as part of her meal. Since she cannot chew, I try to veto crackers. But she insisted. I told her, "Small bite, Milly." She took a small bite, but within seconds she was gasping. Milly often gets minute pieces of food caught in her windpipe and has to cough them up. There is a danger of aspiration into the lungs and pneumonia, but so far coughing works. On the ship it did not. She could not get the air in that would enable her to expel the food.

We were lunching with a British couple we'd met. They looked panicked. I said, feigning jauntiness, "Sorry, this happens," and jumped up. I ran behind Milly and lifted her around the torso, jerking hard on her abdomen. The cracker came out quickly. After Milly got her breath, she insisted on continuing lunch. I said, "No more crackers, Milly. Ever." She does not obey the rule.

The second Heimlich came three months later. Our friends Bob and Phyllis Greenberger—he of the *Wall Street Journal*, and she the head of the Society for Women's Health Research—always host a black-tie New Year's Eve party packed with Washington journalists and political activists, with a sprinkling of liberal congressmen and State Department officials. But so many people were out of town for the millennium that Bob and Phyllis held a costume party in the early spring instead. Our original plan was that Milly would go as FDR and I as Eleanor. I managed to find a getup for her, but not for myself, so I uncreatively just bought a Richard Nixon mask. We were sitting with the Siegels before dinner. I went off to refill our Cokes, and when I got back Mark was saying, "Milly needs help." She had tried to eat a Chinese dumpling. She was gasping and looking panicked. Simultaneously a menacing gurgling sound emanated from her throat.

I thought, "Please, God, no!" and jumped around to the back of her wheelchair. I tried to lift her to a standing position, but I forgot that she was still buckled in. I undid the seatbelt, pulled her up, and began pumping just below her sternum. Mercifully, after two tries, the food popped out. Milly sucked in air for a second, then quickly recovered. I tried to make a joke of it again: "No more dumplings for you! Hummus is all you get." The incident happened so quickly that no one but a horrified Mark Siegel even noticed. I am sure that he could have performed the maneuver in my absence or gotten help from someone else. Milly's "ladies," Grelanda and Felly, know how to do the maneuver, too. Indeed, each has had to do it once.

The third occasion was the scariest. We were at the Siegels' for Thanksgiving dinner. I carefully chopped Milly's turkey and mixed it alternately with stuffing and mashed sweet potatoes. She tried to eat some of it herself, but mostly I guided her fork. Milly seemed to be processing everything smoothly. She took in one forkful of food after another and indicated quickly that she was ready for more. Suddenly she emitted that awful sound, the combination of gasping and gurgling. Everyone at the table, fifteen people, stopped talking and sat stunned and scared. I jumped, wheeled Milly a few feet away from the table, lifted her, and pumped. Nothing came out. I did it again, and nothing happened. And again. I prayed. I had a fleeting vision of an ambulance arriving, a rescue squad, an emergency room, and possible brain damage, Milly living on a respirator. On the fifth or sixth try, though, the food began to come up. But Milly continued to choke, so I repeated the procedure. More food came out. And more. As it turned out, much of her meal had gone down her windpipe, not her esophagus. And worst of all, she hadn't known it was happening. This could happen again at any time, with disastrous consequences. Thankfully, it has not.

Even though she is supposed to stick to soft foods, Milly always wants to violate the rule, and it's impossible not to accede to her wishes sometimes. She insists on getting popcorn at the movies, for instance. I order it heavily buttered to make it softer, but often she makes disturbing coughing sounds as she eats it. I whisper in the dark at least once per show to ask if she needs the Heimlich. She has never needed more than a sip of Diet Coke to wash the popcorn down. Since the last Heimlich we have worked it out that if she does require help she's to wave a fist at me. Fortunately, she hasn't had to.

But I'm always scared that something will stick in her throat that the person with her can't dislodge, or that Milly will try to eat something she shouldn't when the person is out walking the dog or running an errand. In my worst fantasy I come back to find Milly choking, fail at Heimlich, call 911, and wait an eternity for help while trying CPR. If this happened, Milly could die in my arms, or if emergency crews did arrive, her brain could be deprived of oxygen long enough to put her into a coma. Then I would be faced with the decision about whether to leave her in a vegetative state.

That terrible fate is the worst possible future that Milly and I face. But it is probably not the likeliest, which is terrible enough. It is that three months, six months, or a year from now, Milly will be unable to swallow anything. There are moments already when even ice cream or applesauce goes down her windpipe, causing her to choke and gag. At such times I fear that we will have to decide soon whether to have her fed through a tube surgically implanted into her stomach. Presumably she will be alert and able to tell me, one way or the other, what she wants. I can imagine that she will be ambivalent, part of her wanting to die, part afraid to die, part wanting to live. Would she look to me to decide? What would I say? Surely I will say—indeed, I have said—that she should stay alive. We could convert our second bedroom into a hospital room if necessary.

But later, after months on a feeding tube, Milly will surely despair and say that she wants it removed. I can imagine her wanting that one day and becoming doubtful the next. It's also conceivable that someday she will be utterly unable to communicate, as happened to Mo Udall and to Milly herself at NIH when her body was deprived of L-dopa. As with the loved ones of Mo

Udall, who died in 1999, I may not know what Milly wants or whether she retains the mental capacity to want anything. What should I do? Could I order the tube's removal and watch Milly starve to death? Now, I think I could. But in fact, I may lack the courage. Or I may be so guilty about wishing for the end to our ordeal that I find myself prolonging it. I will surely ask God what to do.

This is not the way I want this story to end. I want a medical miracle to save her. But even if there is none, our story will not end. However I lose Milly, if I lose Milly, memory will survive. I remember the restaurant where we met, the raincoat she was wearing the moment I knew I had fallen in love with her, the soft couch where we first made love, the smell and the taste of her, the ski slope breakup. I remember everything about the day and night we were restored to each other for keeps—the beach, the Beatles, the pot, the rainstorm, and the kisses under a street lamp. And thirty-four years of marriage—the fighting, the children, her steel, her generosity. Her courage. I will keep working to end Parkinson's disease on her behalf, and I will hug her in my heart forever.

2002 *Afterword*

⌁⌁⌁ In the late spring of 2001, just as *Saving Milly* was about to be published, the life-or-death "feeding tube decision" I so dreaded suddenly rushed upon us. Milly was nearly unable to swallow anything—food, liquids, or medicine. A simple meal of soup or oatmeal took hours to complete, and Milly's distress at not being able to eat made swallowing solid foods even more difficult. We shifted to Ensure and other supplements, but she also had difficulty drinking and pulling liquids up through a straw.

She subsisted largely on a blended-and-frozen mixture of Ensure, ice cream, and fruit, which she was able to swallow better than anything else—though not in sufficient volume to give her adequate nutrition. And she was getting less than optimal doses of Sinemet and her other medicines.

These combined deprivations left her weak much of the time. She couldn't help lift herself out of a chair, and her legs could barely support her when I tried to "dance" her from room to room. Also, she suffered some scary near-fainting incidents. In mid-May, a week or so before the book was scheduled to be unveiled at the Udall dinner, Milly's friend Jill Schuker and her caregiver Grelanda Te called me at work to say that Milly's face had gone deathly pale and that, while conscious, she was unable to respond to them.

I called Milly's neurology nurse, Marge Gillespie, who said they should lie her down and elevate her legs. She also said that the decision about whether Milly would accept a feeding tube could not be put off much longer. I called home. Jill said they'd already done what Marge advised and that Milly seemed okay. But I knew that Marge was right.

For months, I had avoided discussing the issue with Milly. I feared she would follow through on her vow to refuse a feeding tube and starve to death. She had enshrined this wish in her living will. As I hung up with Marge, I had the fleeting dread that instead of enjoying the launch of this book together, Milly and I would spend the coming weeks in a hospice awaiting her death. I planned to argue for the tube—and, if necessary, beg her to take it—but I couldn't be sure what Milly would do.

Thankfully, Milly decided to live. And the resolution of the issue was infinitely easier than I had envisioned. Sometime amid the blur of events in May and June—I cannot remember exactly when—I simply blurted out to Milly, "You have to decide about the feeding tube soon." So many good things were happening at the time—Andréa's medical school graduation, book parties, a cover story about us in USA Today—that I hoped Milly would decide to live and enjoy them. When I broached the subject, she said, "I'll do it." "You'll have a tube installed? You'll stick around?" I asked. "Yes," she said. It seemed no big thing to her. But to me, it was the world.

Installation of a PEG tube is surprisingly simple. PEG stands for percutaneous endoscopic gastronomy, which means it's a "through the skin, installed using a camera, into the stomach" tube. It's done on an out-patient basis with a local anesthetic and mild sedation. Milly had the operation on July 25. It took no more than 20 minutes. The surgeon passed a tube down Milly's throat and into her stomach. It had a tiny camera and very bright light on the end that showed him where to make a small incision on the outside of her abdomen. He inserted the end of a plastic tube and inflated a little balloon inside her stomach to hold the tube in place. Then he bandaged the wound and called Grelanda and me into the recovery room to show us how to use the tube and keep it clean. He prescribed an antibiotic to prevent infection and gave us an ointment to apply until the wound healed. That was it.

Ever since, eight or so times a day, Grelanda, Milly's other caregiver, Felly Relano, or I open the cap at the end of the tube, insert a plastic syringe, and pour in Milly's medicines, crushed and dissolved in water, or a vitamin-rich liquid food formula called Jevity Plus. Diet Sprite, Milly's favorite drink, keeps the tube clean. Obviously, though, she can't taste it. Typically, Milly was concerned whether the tube, 16 inches long, would cause a noticeable bulge in her clothing. Looped and taped to her tummy, it doesn't.

Ensuring her adequate nutrition, hydration, and medication, the tube had an immediate positive effect on Milly's strength and spirits. Episodes of near-fainting and low blood pressure stopped. More gradually, she has become better able to walk and stand with assistance. And, she says that she wanted to live.

I fancied—until recently—that all the excitement connected

with publication of the book had motivated Milly's decision to live. Certainly it was buoying to both of us. First, the *Washington Post* magazine published an excerpt, causing people to walk up to us on the street and tell us how inspiring we were. We started getting letters from around the country when Susan Page wrote her *USA Today* piece, which was accompanied by a huge picture of us on the front page. At one book party, a dozen or so of Milly's former clients showed up and told her again how she'd helped them change their lives. Our daughters made moving speeches about how ours was the most successful marriage they'd ever encountered or could hope to. Alex made a short video from our collection of home movies that was played at the Udall dinner and again when I was invited to appear on NBC's *Today Show*. I also was interviewed on C-SPAN's *Booknotes*, practically every program on the Fox News Channel, and on dozens of other TV and radio shows.

Reviews of the book were sometimes dazzling. Andrew Ferguson, in the *Wall Street Journal*, wrote that "it is one of those uncommon books that manages—quietly, beyond any expectation—to ennoble its author and its readers alike." The *Chicago Tribune's* reviewer said it was "unflinching, honest, powerful, unvarnished, heartrending." Others said it was "a beautiful love letter," "tender, loving, and funny," and "a truly compelling read." The *New York Times* said it was "excruciatingly painful," but also "a powerful argument for more financing for Parkinson's research." There was hardly a negative word.

The book came out just as President Bush was going through his own excruciating process of deciding whether to allow federal funding of medical research using stem cells derived from (and requiring the destruction of) fertilized human embryos. Parkinson's is one of the diseases that may be cured someday through stem cell research. Milly and I appeared on ABC's *Nightline* amid the controversy. The *Washington Post* columnist Richard Cohen wrote that "if George W. Bush reads just one book this summer, I hope it's *Saving Milly*." He said, "I finished it last night in tears." Such publicity and gracious words helped land the book on some national bestseller lists.

The most gratifying—and daunting—response we got, however, was the mail. Hundreds of people wrote to offer Milly and me encouragement and prayers. Some were victims of Parkinson's or other chronic diseases, some the spouses of victims, recounting their own medical and spiritual journeys or telling us how our story had inspired them to persevere. Others recommended alternative medical treatments for Parkinson's. We received so many letters that I was unable to respond to them. I think about the unanswered mail almost daily, with guilt.

But to my even deeper regret, the book caused pain to Milly's wonderful foster family in Chicago. I could not have avoided writing that one of the houses Milly grew up in was infested with bedbugs. She is convinced that soaking her mattress and bedroom walls with DDT to kill them somehow triggered her Parkinson's. However, my account left out the fact that the Villarreal family swept and scrubbed the house constantly to keep it clean. Members of the family told me that they, their friends, and some business associates felt that I'd portrayed the home as "filthy" and the neighborhood as a "slum." Moreover, they said, I conveyed a sense that Milly's childhood was unrelievedly miserable, leaving out joyful times—hayrides, birthdays, pranks, and graduations. In writing disparagingly about Milly's nephew, who once lived with us, I also neglected to say that Alex and Andréa loved him as they would an older brother, and still do.

I am deeply sorry for the hurt I caused—particularly because the book came out just as Milly's valiant foster mother, Annie, was dying from respiratory problems. She spent weeks in the hospital, with family members led by Milly's sister, Lori, standing twenty-four-hour watch as she sometimes rallied, neared death, and rallied again until her system finally failed in late July. Annie evidently shared the family's dismay with the book, even though I'd written that she was the person who'd given Milly her values, her self-confidence, and her giant capacity for love. Milly and I scheduled flights to Chicago to see her, but had to cancel each time because Annie was in a medical crisis. We saw her last at her wake, attended by hundreds of people she'd helped in Chicago's Mexican-American community, plus local and national politicians. Thankfully, most members of the family acted as though my book had never been written.

While the feeding tube improved Milly's health and strength, it did not have much effect on her ability to communicate. Various book reviewers wrote that ours had been a "tempestuous" or "volatile" marriage. I think those words imply infidelity and separations, which never occurred. A better way to describe our marriage, pre-Parkinson's, is "loud." We argued a lot and we didn't keep our voices down. But in recent years, as Milly's disease has progressed, our marriage has gone virtually silent. In the morning before I leave for work and when I get home at night, I tell Milly what I've been doing and what I'm thinking. I tell her often that I love her. But we don't have real conversations.

In a cruelty akin to Beethoven's deafness, Parkinson's has robbed this gifted therapist and wise friend of her ability to question, penetrate, and give advice. Milly tries to speak, but most of the time she cannot enunciate words clearly enough to be understood. She also has lost the manual dexterity needed to punch computer keys or point to letters on a chart to spell out words.

This makes communication arduous and its level has become mostly very simple. Grelanda invented the catchphrase we use when Milly is trying to say something: "What's the topic, Milly?" It usually has to do with calling our girls, movies we're going to see, her clothing choices, or the fact she's out of spending money.

One small miracle I'd hoped for didn't occur, but another may be in process. NIH experiments with yohimbine, a drug derived from an old African aphrodisiac, have not succeeded in helping Milly speak. The drug raised Milly's voice volume once, when administered intravenously, then failed to do so again. Doses administered through the feeding tube made her body shake, caused drooling, and gave her the hiccups, but had no effect on her speech.

Believe it or not, though, we've recently achieved successful results with Godiva white chocolate bars, which I now buy in bulk and which Milly can swallow. I have no idea what ingredient in the candy stimulates her voice, but there is no mistaking the effect. Sometimes she can be heard.

And so, we've begun to talk more. She still cannot form words well, so I have to stop her and ask the topic or say, "Slow down. What's the first word, Milly?" When I understand that, we slowly work through her sentence. I ask her to spell words I can't make out. Eventually, her thoughts come through. And some of them are moving. Preparing this afterword, I asked her why she had decided last year to live. Did the book influence her? "No," she said. "I just decided to live." I asked about it another time and she said, "I decided to stay alive because I have you to love."

Just before Christmas—about the time we were transitioning from yohimbine to Godiva—I also asked her about God. She said, "I love God. I talk to Him every day. I pray for you and for the girls. I ask Him to give me my speech back." Stunned, I asked her when she had stopped believing that God had abandoned her. She said it was last year, when I stopped writing on Sundays and we started going back to church regularly—and when, she said, the priests at St. Columba's began coming to where we sit in church and praying over her at communion time. Every week this gesture brings tears to my eyes because it has had such an impact on Milly. I asked her again recently why she had changed her mind about God. "He is the only one I can talk to whenever I want," she said. I am profoundly grateful that Milly is spiritually at peace. It is the fulfillment of many of my own prayers.

Some elements of what I called in the book "God's work"— medical research—are proceeding. President Bush, prodded by Senators Tom Harkin of Iowa and Arlen Specter of Pennsylvania, is fulfilling his promise to complete the process of doubling the NIH budget over a five-year period. On the other hand, he failed for more than a year to appoint an NIH director, leaving the agency without effective leadership.

And, despite the urging of disease groups—led by the Juvenile Diabetes Research Foundation, the Parkinson's Action Network, and the Christopher Reeve Paralysis Foundation—Bush decided to permit only limited federal funding of embryonic stem cell research. To the good, he did not ban it entirely, but decided to fund only research using cells already derived on the day of his decision, August 9, 2001. He claimed that some sixty "lines"—or batches—of cells were available for research around the world. But many scientists dispute the number and contend that Bush's decision means that private funds and scientists in other countries will have to carry the research forward. The president also wants to make it illegal to clone embryos to acquire stem cells for research and therapeutic purposes.

One group that will vigorously advance stem cell and other promising Parkinson's research is the Michael J. Fox Foundation. Powered by Michael's dedication and endearing nature, the foundation attracted a first-rate board of directors, scientific advisory panel and staff, and raised more than $11 million in its first full year of operation. The foundation has conducted three research initiatives, attracting hundreds of grant applications from scientists around the world—proving, in case anyone doubted it, that impressive strides can be made in curing Parkinson's if adequate funding is available. In its first two years, the Fox Foundation may have raised as much as $30 million and lead half a dozen major new research initiatives.

Besides leading the foundation, Michael has written a wonderful book, *Lucky Man*, in which he says that he would not trade the life he has had with Parkinson's for the one he might have had without it. The sentiment only deepens my devotion to Michael, but I cannot share it for Milly and me. I would give anything for her not to have Parkinson's disease, regardless of where that might have led our lives.

At best, the Fox Foundation and other private groups can fund only a fraction of the research possible for the federal government. The NIH says it is now spending $155.9 million per year on Parkinson's, or about $156 per U.S. victim. This figure includes both direct and "related" projects, so it does not mean that funding has been quintupled since 1994, when the Parkinson's Action Network began demonstrating how underfunded PD research was in comparison to other diseases.

Prodded by Congress, NIH conducted a study in 1999 to determine what the optimum level of PD funding would be. The study confirmed scientists' testimony that promising strides could be made in gene and stem cell therapies, surgery, neuron repair, epidemiology, and prevention. And it said that one billion additional dollars could be spent productively on PD research over five years, beginning with $70 million in the first year. Alas, despite the best efforts of a rejuvenated Parkinson's Action Network, that money has not been asked for by the executive branch nor appropriated by Congress, although it's been pushed for hard by some members, notably Senator Harkin. Joan Samuelson remains the president and guiding spirit of PAN, but now she has a vigorous board, executive director, and advocacy director working with her, increasingly making PAN the Washington voice of a united Parkinson's disease community.

There continues to be every reason to believe that a cure for Parkinson's will be discovered within five or ten years, but it also remains true that—barring a miracle—it will not arrive in time to save Milly, particularly because she suffers from a complicated case. Thanks to her inner will and the grace of God, Milly has decided to remain alive and to fight Parkinson's to the finish. She has revised her living will to give her the option—or me, as her agent, in the event she is totally incapacitated and unable to communicate—of discontinuing feeding and liquids. But her rate of decline has slowed, so that decision is probably years away.

I will do everything in my power to make her life worth living. To the extent what I do is work, it is never hard work and it is always lightened by love. Milly has recovered some of her ability to swallow, for instance, and so I delight in buying expensive ice cream for her and cooking tubs of vichyssoise almost as rich as ice cream. I do not have infinite patience trying to divine what she is saying, one word or one letter at a time, but I always want to know what she wants and thinks, whether it's mundane or profound. I shout at her when she tries to do something unsafe, like trying to get out of bed when no one's in the room to help. But I also admire her courage. I do wish I had someone to have intimate conversations with. I wish I had more time to play tennis and golf and read books, but there is nothing I would rather do than sit or lie next to Milly, hold her hand and kiss her. I tell her she is beautiful. She winces at herself in the mirror and says that Parkinson's has made her ugly. But it hasn't. Each time I look at her, my heart melts. I still do not know how this story ends. Thankfully, it is not ending soon.

Index

Saving Milly

Love, Politics, and Parkinson's Disease

MORTON KONDRACKE

A Reader's Guide

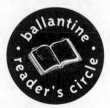

A Conversation with Morton Kondracke

Fred Barnes is *executive editor of* The Weekly Standard, *and Morton Kondracke's co-host on the Fox News Channel political show* The Beltway Boys.

Fred Barnes: What was Milly's reaction to your book?

Morton Kondracke: Milly read the chapters as they were being written, then I read it to her right after the book came out, and again recently. The best thing she said was, "This is a great love story." The first time she read the last chapter she said it depressed her. It is sad. It's about death and about losing Milly.

FB: What effect did the book have on Milly?

MK: The book helped change the ending, I think. Partly because of the hoopla connected with the book—the praise it got, the publicity, having her picture on the front page of *USA Today*, and the hundreds of letters we received—she was encouraged to get a feeding tube. I think Milly, being the indomitable person she is, probably would have decided to stay alive under any circumstances. But the book has made her life more exciting.

FB: Do you have any regrets about revealing intimate details of your marriage with utmost candor?

MK: I don't. I didn't reveal *every* intimate detail about our marriage or what the illness involves, about what Milly can't do now and what I do to help her. I did tell a lot because I figured this was the only biography that would ever be written about either of us, so I should tell as much of the truth as I could about our lives. And I wanted people to understand in detail what a wretched disease Parkinson's is so they'd help us fight for a cure.

FB: While writing the book, did you ever pause and think, "Maybe I shouldn't be revealing this"?

MK: There were a couple of minor things that my daughters, Alexandra and Andréa, asked me to take out and I did.

FB: What did Alexandra and Andréa think about the book? And what effect did it have on your family?

MK: They are very proud of me for having written it and happy about its success. It's helped draw us even closer together. Friends threw two wonderful book parties in Washington. At one of them, both of my daughters spoke very movingly of their love and admiration for Milly—about what a strong mother she is and how much courage she's shown. They said that ours was the best marriage they'd ever encountered or could imagine. They were both eloquent. I was very proud of them. They say they learned things from the book about Milly's upbringing that they hadn't focused on, though I don't think they were surprised by anything. Right before the book came out, Alex found boxes of old home movies we'd taken and prepared a video that was played on television a couple of times when I was interviewed. She said she learned from those movies what a stylish, "hip" person Milly was in the old days.

FB: If you could write the book again, are there things you'd put in that you didn't?

MK: One thing for sure. Members of Milly's foster family in Chicago were deeply hurt by the implication that they were not only poor, but didn't keep their house clean. And also by the impression that Milly's childhood was totally miserable. Neither is correct, and I'd try to make it clear that they scrubbed a lot. But their house was old and it had bedbugs that couldn't be cleaned away—hence the use of DDT that Milly thinks triggered her Parkinson's. Also, though her mother abandoned her and her father died when she was young, I tried to say that she was raised by a wonderful family, the Villarreals, who gave her great values and inner strength. Milly feels nothing but gratitude toward them, and so do I. So I'd write more about good times in her childhood.

FB: Your book got some phenomenal reviews and sold well. Was this what you expected? Were there any disappointments?

MK: I had so much favorable feedback from friends before the book came out that I hoped it would be well received. What happened was beyond all my expectations—some amazingly laudatory reviews and a lot of publicity that happened partly because President Bush's decision was pending on federal funding of embryonic stem cell research. *Saving Milly* made it onto two national bestseller lists. And the mail has not stopped, especially from people sharing their own experiences with chronic illness. Of course, once you get a taste of success like this, you don't know the limits and you lose your objectivity. So you hope that maybe you've written another *Tuesdays with Morrie*, and there's a letdown when you realize you haven't. I was disappointed by a few friends in the media who I thought would pay attention to the book and didn't. For a while I was also disappointed that I didn't get to appear on the *Oprah Winfrey Show*, this being a story about courage and commitment. Then, when Michael J. Fox's book came out, I did get invited. So overwhelmingly I'm gratified by the response.

FB: You've said that both psychotherapy and your religious faith helped you handle Milly's illness. Did they conflict or complement each other?

MK: No, they didn't conflict. I suppose some psychotherapists see religion as too rigid and absolute and some religious people think therapy means "whatever makes you happy." But as I've experienced therapy and faith, they're entirely compatible. Religion is all about ends and ultimate things—your relationship to the greatest power in the universe and whether you've enlisted in the army that fights for Truth, Goodness, Beauty, and Love. Psychotherapy is more about means—improving your capacity for love, openness, and generosity. I think a good therapist can be an angel, doing God's work. Mine, Dr. Dorree Lynn, is. And her message is strikingly similar to that of your and my spiritual adviser, Jerry Leachman, who preaches out of the Bible the importance of having a grateful heart—realizing that all you have is a gift from God. Dorree, when I'm inclined to dismiss the good things in my life and concentrate on what I don't have, tells me that's sacrilegious. The two of them are entirely in sync and I'm happy for it.

FB: Why did you need psychotherapy in the first place?

MK: I have a natural tendency to be moderately depressed. I wasn't very trusting, was closed to other people and self-absorbed, narcissistic and judgmental. Maybe you can pray your way out of such things, but I think God's answer would be to send a friend or a therapist to help you. I've had both—a therapist who helped me name and work out my psychological bad habits, and generous friends who taught me how to be more generous. In Milly, I've had both a therapist and a friend. I can't say I'm fully where I ought to be even yet. Everything is a work-in-progress.

FB: Why did you need your Christian faith?

MK: I've always believed in God and I was brought up in the Christian tradition. Milly's illness has made me more dependent on God—utterly dependent, in fact. I say "God, I need your help" about twenty times a day. And He does help me. The important process for me now is trying to mature as a Christian. As I wrote in the book, I believe completely in Jesus' message. I'm studying his message and his life more deeply, but I still don't have the same connection that I feel with God.

FB: Some of your friends, including me, believe you were too hard on yourself in describing "the old Mort" as self-centered and snobbish before Milly's illness. What do you say about that?

MK: I don't think I was a monster, but I certainly had chronic flaws. I may have played them up to contrast myself with Milly, who was and is the opposite of all I was—generous, forthright, utterly democratic and unimpressed by status, and pretty fearless. I may have emphasized my weaknesses to underline her strengths, but I didn't distort anything.

FB: Your old friend, Michael Kinsley, the editor of Slate.com, revealed in *Time* magazine last December that he has Parkinson's and said he chose "denial" as a strategy, telling very few people and continuing his life as usual. You and Milly chose what he calls "confrontation." Why?

MK: I've known Michael Kinsley for twenty-five years. He was my editor at *The New Republic*. I'd learned from others a few years ago that he had Parkinson's. I was relieved when he stopped keeping it secret. Psychologically, Milly and I did try to practice denial for about a year. We didn't conceal her tentative diagnosis, but we did try to deny it to ourselves and try to find an alternative diagnosis. Milly is such an up-front person that she doesn't have much capacity for secrecy and deception. She didn't tell her psychotherapy clients right away, but she did tell everyone else. I followed her lead. If it had been up to me, or if it had been my illness, I might have opted for a third option Kinsley describes—acceptance. But Milly's distress was so great that I couldn't do that. And I don't have much capacity for secrecy and deception, either. Kinsley disparages what he calls "aggressive victimhood," which he says is socially trendy. Michael is such a contrarian and ironist that whatever society favors is what he won't do. But aggressive victims and their families are indispensable in getting more research money for Parkinson's and other diseases. So I hope now that Michael Kinsley will join us.

FB: You've lobbied the White House and Congress for more funding for medical research. You almost lost your press credentials. How did you resolve this dispute?

MK: I resolved it by obeying the rules of the congressional press galleries and giving up the chairmanship of a group called NIH2. It was moribund anyway, and the cause of doubling the NIH budget was succeeding, so obeying the ethics police was easy. On the larger issue, "should journalists ever lobby?" I agree in principle that they shouldn't. On the other hand, I don't regret what I did. I thought my wife's life was on the line and I had to do whatever I could. Parkinson's disease research is still deeply underfunded, and lobbying Congress to change that is still necessary. I don't do it myself, but I help the Parkinson's Action Network do so and I speak out at every opportunity, which is within the rules.

FB: Milly receives medical treatment at the National Institutes of Health free of charge while you continue to campaign for

doubling the NIH's budget. Isn't there a conflict of interest there?

MK: I don't feel any conflict at all. I would support doubling NIH's budget even if Milly weren't receiving care there. And Milly's been willing to be a guinea pig whenever NIH has asked her to join in a clinical trial. I acknowledge we have received far more from NIH than we've given back. If it were legally possible for me to pay for her care there, I would. Or, my insurance would. And, I've been critical of NIH, too, especially its reluctance to a fight an all-out war on Parkinson's.

FB: Why does it do that?

MK: It is determined not to "play favorites" among diseases, even though NIH itself says that Parkinson's is the most curable of all neurodegenerative diseases.

FB: How has the political community responded to the effort to double NIH's budget?

MK: Pretty well. The initial impetus for doing this came from Congress, particularly from Senators Tom Harkin of Iowa and Arlen Specter of Pennsylvania, among those currently in office. Increases of 13, 14, or 15 percent have been approved for four years, a pace that would produce a doubling over five or six years. The Bush administration supports doubling over five years, but Bush is playing favorites on behalf of cancer and, of course, bioterrorism research. The big question is, "What happens next?" If we return to increases of 5 percent or less per year—which I fear Bush's budget people favor—it will be a disaster, like hitting the brakes on a fast-moving vehicle. Labs will have to close, projects will be stopped, and people will get fired. Disease cures will be delayed. A lot of thought needs to be given to what happens after doubling.

FB: You argued that President Bush should permit broad use of stem cell research on so-called "leftover" embryos at fertilization clinics. How do you feel about "cloning," or creating fertilized embryos for research purposes? Any doubts about that?

MK: Actually, I am torn about the cloning issue. I'm definitely against cloning to produce babies, which has all kinds of "brave new world" implications, as well as being dangerous. In animals, many clones have terrible birth defects. On the other hand, so-called "therapeutic cloning" has great advantages. People could contribute cells from their own bodies, have embryos cloned, and use the resulting stem cells to repair defective parts without tissue-rejection problems. But, there is a slippery slope problem here: if it's okay to create embryos and extract stem cells when they are five or six days old, why not let them grow five or six months and "farm" fetuses for hearts and other body organs—also to save lives? Frankly, I hope this moral dilemma can be avoided by the success of research on adult stem cells derived from blood, marrow, or even fat cells and require no cloning. If I were in Congress, I guess I'd vote to allow therapeutic cloning, but limit research to days-old embryos.

FB: **Why does it take celebrities such as you and Michael J. Fox to stir public interest in a disease such as Parkinson's?**

MK: We live in a publicity-minded culture and celebrities attract more publicity than anyone else—especially if they are as legitimately beloved as Michael J. Fox and Muhammad Ali are. Members of Congress are close to the most publicity-minded group in America, always looking for witnesses who'll attract TV cameras to their hearings and attention to themselves. But celebrity hasn't been enough to win the fight for adequate Parkinson's money, at least not yet. What it really takes is a powerful politician who is dedicated to the cause.

FB: **Has the warfare among disease groups for federal money persisted?**

MK: No, the fact that the NIH budget is doubling has significantly reduced the competition. In fact, the major disease groups have collaborated wonderfully in this common effort. But the competition will start again if, God forbid, the budgets begin to go flat again. Nobody will say openly "Cut cancer and give to us" or "Cut AIDS," but they will be inclined to stop cooperating and just go for themselves.

FB: Do you plan another book?

MK: I think there is a useful book to be written about dysfunction—you might say, civil war—in the American health system. We have the best health care in the world, but it is much less good than it could be, largely because cost pressures are threatening quality. Everybody's fighting—doctors against insurance companies and HMOs, hospitals with their own nurses, malpractice lawyers with all providers, the government with drug companies. Through Medicare and Medicaid, the government sets prices for most medical procedures and the process is horribly inefficient. And then there's the growing problem of the uninsured, who often don't get attention until they are sick enough to go to an emergency room. All this could be described in a compelling way, and I have some ideas about solutions. I think health care will be back as a major national issue and perhaps I could help the process.

FB: So you'd go from *Saving Milly* to *Saving Health Care*?

MK: I'm looking for a better title, thanks.

Reading Group Questions and Topics for Discussion

1. How do you personally reconcile the existence of evil in the world with the idea of an all-powerful, all-knowing, and loving God? Why do you think bad things happen to good people?

2. How would you react if you were diagnosed with a chronic, incurable illness, or if this happened to a person you love? Would your reaction be more like Mort's or Milly's?

3. The journalist Michael Kinsley, announcing in *Time* magazine that he has Parkinson's, defended the idea of "denial"—keeping the disease secret for as long as possible and trying to get on with one's life. He disparaged "aggressive victimhood" or "confrontation"—in other words, going public and demanding action. What would your choice be?

4. Why do you suppose that women are so much more likely to "stick it out" with a chronically ill spouse than men are?

5. Should government—federal, state, or local—provide assistance (whether in money or nursing services) to spouses caring for a chronically ill mate?

6. Does it strike you as unethical for a journalist to lobby the White House or Congress for what he or she believes is a good cause?

7. How did you react to the fact that wide disparities—by hundreds, sometimes even thousands of dollars per victim—exist in federal research funding for various diseases? How do you think federal dollars should be allocated?

8. Should allocations of disease research money be "political"? Can it be otherwise as long as Congress appropriates the money for medical research?

9. Would you favor creating a dependable, dedicated money source for medical research, such as a 1 percent or 2 percent tax on health insurance premiums or a tax increase on such illness-producing products as tobacco, alcohol, or high-fat foods?

10. Do you believe that human embryos "leftover" at fertility clinics and destined to be discarded should be used to extract stem cells for medical research? If so, should the federal government fund this research?

11. Should the government outlaw the cloning of human embryos for both reproductive and research purposes, as President Bush advocates?

12. Should terminally ill people have the right to end their own lives? If so, under what circumstances? In hospices, where they can be kept comfortable as they refuse food and water? Or by assisted suicide, in which a doctor actually administers lethal drugs?

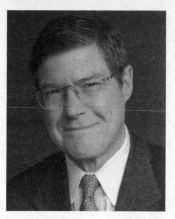

About the Author

MORTON KONDRACKE was for many years a regular panelist on *The McLaughlin Group* and is currently a regular contributor for the Fox News Channel and co-host of its weekly political show, *The Beltway Boys*, executive editor and columnist for the Capitol Hill newspaper *Roll Call*, and a semi-regular commentator on *Fox News Sunday*. He is a board member of both the Parkinson's Action Network and the Michael J. Fox Foundation for Parkinson's Research. He lives in Washington, D.C.